LA GOULUE

THE QUEEN OF THE MOULIN ROUGE

Her Story

LA GOULUE

THE QUEEN OF THE MOULIN ROUGE

Her Story

MARYLINE MARTIN

Translated by Leonard Rosmarin

mosaic PRESS

Library and Archives Canada Cataloguing in Publication

Title: The Queen of the Moulin Rouge : her story / by Maryline Martin; translated by Leonard Rosmarin.

Other titles: Goulue. English

Names: Martin, Maryline (Author), author. | Rosmarin, Léonard A., translator.

Description: Translation of: La Goulue, reine du Moulin Rouge.

Identifiers: Canadiana (print) 20210211776
Canadiana (ebook) 20210211857

ISBN 9781771615884 (softcover) ISBN 9781771615891 (PDF)
ISBN 9781771615907 (EPUB) ISBN 9781771615914 (Kindle)

Subjects: LCSH: Goulue, 1866-1929. | LCSH: Moulin-Rouge (Night club : Paris, France)—

History—19th century. | LCSH: Moulin-Rouge (Night club : Paris, France)—History—20th century. | LCSH: Dancers—France—Paris—Biography. | LCSH: Women dancers—France —Paris—Biography. | LCSH: Paris (France)—Social life and customs—19th century. | LCSH: Paris (France)—Social life and customs—20th century. LCGFT: Biographies.

Classification: LCC GV1785.G68 M3713 2021
DDC 792.7092—dc23

All rights reserved. Without limiting the rights under copyright reserved here, no part of this publicationm ay be reproduced, stored in or introduced into any retrieval system, or transmitted in any form or by any means—electronic, mechanical, by photocopy, recording or otherwise—without the prior written permission and consent of both the copyright owners and the Publisher of this book.
All materials in this book are published on a non-exclusive basis.

Published by Mosaic Press, Oakville, Ontario, Canada, 2021.

MOSAIC PRESS, Publishers
www.Mosaic-Press.com
English Copyright © Mosaic Press, 2021, Translated by Leonard Rosmarin
Originally Published in French | La Goulue: Reine du Moulin Rouge
© Editions du Rocher, 2019

Printed and bound in Canada.

ONTARIO ARTS COUNCIL
CONSEIL DES ARTS DE L'ONTARIO
an Ontario government agency
un organisme du gouvernement de l'Ontario

Funded by the Government of Canada
Financé par le gouvernement du Canada

Canada

ONTARIO CREATES

MOSAIC PRESS
1252 Speers Road, Units 1 & 2, Oakville, Ontario, L6L 5N9
(905) 825-2130 • info@mosaic-press.com • www.mosaic-press.com

We're going to run, to go out
Out on foot... not in a berlin!
We'll reveal no more than a glimpse
Of what is above the boot.
Ah! What a fuss, what coquettish care,
What hard work for the chambermaid!
Finally, it is done, she appears
The Parisienne armed for war!
On seeing her, they go crazy
And feel something pounding right there.
Her dress goes swish, swish, swish
With her nose in the wind, scurrying, scurrying, scurrying
She goes on straight ahead.
When they cross her path, each passerby
Stops and says: "God! How beautiful she is!"

La Vie Parisienne (Paris Life), *Act III,*
"We're gong to run, to go out," Jacques Offenbach

***

"My dear, yesterday I met a woman whom I did not know. I invited her to supper... She devoured everything. –Ah, no doubt she was La Goulue..." *Le Sphinx*, October 24, 1885.

****

"A bouquet of living, pearly orchids blooms in an absinth dawn. A carnal palpitation rose up from among the lacework and smoky stockings..." Armand Leroux (*L'Intransigeant*, 1956)

TABLE OF CONTENTS

FOREWORD

La Goulue has for a long time been considered a rotten person devoid of intelligence. An opinion which does not correspond to the reality of the archives and which I wished to make public with this biography.

My research led to a meeting with Jean-Luc Pehau-Ricau, Director of Public Relations at the Moulin Rouge. On a spring evening he opened up for me the doors of this mythical place that celebrated its 130 years in 2019. He shared a treasure with me: the intimate diary of Louise that I have been able to read through and study with deep emotion.

Mme Isabelle Ducatez, the Director of the Historical and Archeological Society of the 9th and 18th Paris and Old Montmartre districts, also allowed me access to a magnificent collection of photos, newspapers, magazines…

Bringing together these different sources enabled me to put into place, one by one, the pieces for the portrait of a very modern woman.

I also wished to bring back to life two people who were by La Goulue's side: Pierre Lazareff and Jean Marèze (the brother of Francis Carco). Both were journalists at *Paris-Midi* then at *Paris-Soir* and devoted many pages to the Queen of the Moulin Rouge. In their column dedicated to "Celebrities of Yesterday and Today," these two people to whom she referred affectionately as "her little biographers" supported her until her sad end on January 29, 1929.

I have taken the liberty to imagine what Jean Marèse could have written. This, then, is the only flight of imagination I have allowed myself in the prologue (*Behind The Scenes at Paris-Midi*), the entr'acte and epilogue: a few fictitious breaths taken in the breathless destiny of this Magnificent Fishwife…

BEHIND THE SCENES AT *PARIS-MIDI*

I have been locked up in my office now for the past six hours. I have been editing, under diverse and varied pseudonyms, the echoes, theatrical news, faithful and funny reflections coming from the political backstage of the capital, the very stuff that goes into the column *Life in Paris* at *Paris-Midi*[1]. I am waiting impatiently for Pierre Lazareff to call me. Far more than being my boss, he is above all my friend. For him, I am not just the brother of Francis (Carco) but Jeannot. Few people here call me by my real patronym: Jean Marèze. I have not had any news since I left him alone, at Louise's beside. We said goodbye in an oppressive silence. Since then, shaken by the events, I have not been able to write one single suitable sentence about the last play I saw yesterday evening. The wastepaper basket is filled to overflowing with unsuccessful attempts. I am living in another drama, the one involving life. Finally, the telephone ringing fills the space of my retreat. I pick up the receiver. At the other end is Pierrot's nervous voice. His avalanche-like discourse where words overlap one another, and his slight lisp when he speaks too quickly reflect an intense emotion. I light up a Gauloise, more as a reflex than out of need, and learn the unsurprising news: Louise is dead. I stare at the few snowflakes that are whirling around in the frozen Paris air. Again I go through in my mind the events of our morning. Our arrival at Lariboisière. Loulou's weak smile, her hands swollen from water retention. Her messed-up hair lying like a diadem on the pillow. In order not to forget this instant, I engraved in my memory the eagle-like profile and down-turned lips of this dethroned

1. Yves Courrière, *Pierre Lazareff ou le vagabond de l'actualité*, Éditions Gallimard, 1995.

queen of a Paris that no longer existed. A doctor followed by a nurse came up to the sick woman's bed. Reacting to his questioning gaze, Pierrot lied about our identity. We are the only family she has, which is neither entirely true nor entirely false. José, Louise's husband from whom she was separated succumbed to a heart attack in 1915. Simon-Victor, her only son died at the age of 26. Rétoré, her best friend, had remained in Saint-Ouen. He is the one who possesses the duplicates of the keys to her trailer set up at the edge of a vacant lot, on the rue des Entrepôts. As for Pierrot, irresistibly drawn to celebrities of the past and present, he became friends with Louise as of 1923. Out of curiosity, I had followed him till the Tabarin, a Parisian cabaret located at the foot of Montmartre. I remember having been immediately grabbed by the steel blue gaze of this dancer who became a lion tamer, then a candy vendor. As our encounters continued, she nicknamed us affectionately her little biographers… The doctor explained to us why she was hospitalized and seemed pessimistic about a possible recovery. The patient's condition was deteriorating rapidly. After slipping on a frozen sidewalk, Madame Weber lost consciousness, then was admitted to the pneumological department. I don't know how Pierrot had been informed of the accident… The nurse filled a jug of fresh water that she placed on the night table, then took care of another patient. In the early hours of the morning, Louise had asked for a priest. It was time for me to leave. This row of tin beds made me think of a path lined with tombs. The miscreant that I am was completely out of place in this room where the Grim Reaper was intruding little by little. My lips grazed the burning forehead of our friend. While she was murmuring a few words to me, her metallic gaze latched on to me as though she were throwing a bottle out to sea.

I remember leaving Périer Hall like a robber. I carried off with me Louise's last wishes. In the corridor, the arhythmic sound of my footsteps on the marble flagstones brought me back to life little by little. I pulled up the collar of my coat and realized that I had left my scarf on the dying woman's bed. I no longer knew whether I was trembling from fear or cold…

Pierre's silence followed by the clicking of his tongue against his palate evinced his annoyance with my abstracted listening. I feel a bit groggy. My throat is tightening, I am fighting my tears. I have the disagreeable sensation that my clothes are still impregnated with the hospital odor, a mixture of ether, chloroform and death… Pierrot sensed my distress, and confirmed he would arrive shortly. Staring at the silent telephone, with my eyes lost in space, I think again of Louise, her girlish laughter surging out of a body that had become heavy from too much love, too much flesh, too much of everything. Yet they are not all that far away, the moments during which I gathered her memories of the time when she was young and beautiful and would lead the French cancan. By themselves, her words were echoes ready to be printed without any superfluous rewriting.[2]

"You'll tell them, eh, You'll tell them that I was a good girl, my Jeannot?!" That voice coming from beyond the grave was a supplication.

I found again in one of the drawers of my desk the notebook in red moleskin and I sat down in front of my typewriter.

On this 29th of January, 1929, I feel like telling you the story of Louise Weber, better known under the name of La Goulue…

2. *Ibid.*

JOIN IN THE DANCE...

- I -

The home of Madeleine and Dagobert Weber, located at 130, route de la Révolte in Clichy-la-Garenne, was in turmoil. Screams, crying, and snatches of an unknown dialect were issuing from a wide-open window facing a garden planted with trees. The couple originally from Geispolsheim left, in 1860, their little village in the Bas-Rhin region. These two Alsatians did not meet on their home territory but in Clichy. She was a seamstress working from home, he, a carpenter in the new village created by a certain Nicolas Levallois in 1846. They were neighbors, they liked one another, courted one another and agreed that living together would not be such a bad idea since they were crazily in love. Three children later, in 1864, Dagobert would slip the ring on Madeleine's finger for better and for worse...

On the afternoon of July 11, 1866, Amélie, one of the neighbors, came over to help Dagobert run his household. Madeleine had just broken her water, the birth of their fourth child was at hand. Amélie came to prepare the bed, the linen, the fire, the hot water, the thread... Her fingers slipped under the pillow an image of Saint Marguerite who supposedly helped in childbirth.

Dagobert had sent for the midwife, called familiarly "old mother Mandragore", who belonged to a group of twenty thousand women trained and licensed at the time. She had brought Madeleine Eugénie into the world in 1858, who did not survive beyond her first two years, then Marie-Anne in 1861 and Joseph in 1864, the very year the couple decided to get married.

Madeleine was thirty years old. Her body bore the stigmas of her previous pregnancies, but her man still desired her as much as at the start of their relationship with her curves and heavy breasts.

Madeleine was screaming, vociferating, asking that she be freed. Amélie spoke to her softly and made her drink a decoction that would supposedly soothe her and calm her contractions. The future mother struggled but ended up dozing.

The weather was stormy on that day which was two days before the July 14th holiday. Violet clouds obscured the crescent moon, a few lightning flashes tore intermittently through the sky. Far off, the storm was growling. Two moths, drawn to the light, began a dance above the opalines at the risk of burning their wings. Strong odors came up from the garden, entering as the dawn was breaking, a mixture of grass made wet by the rain, and garbage that was rotting in a makeshift shed[1]. Honeysuckle scents refreshed the atmosphere. Pushed by the wind, a window slammed shut. The hot air made the only awning swell up like a boat's sail. Outside some ragpickers were coming out like snails after the rain. With their baskets on their backs, their hooks in one hand, their lanterns in the other, they slid along like phantasmagorical shadows and fought for a few bones with the neighborhood dogs. The pains of giving birth started up again. Madeleine began again to moan and writhe, but old mother Mandragore had arrived. Expert hands pushed against the expectant mother's stomach; the baby was finally in the passage, ready to be born. A cry: the cry of delivery. One can surely recognize a woman giving birth on hearing this sonorous manifestation, as Boccaccio states in the *Decameron*: "Now however comes the moment of birth and the young woman, like all her kind, let out cries." Or Zola: "A loud cry, the furious and triumphant cry of mothers[2].

A brief silence followed by a wail: "It's a girl!"

While cleaning the new-born's body who was already clamouring for her mother's breast, the midwife congratulated Madeleine for her courage. The latter replied that she was happy, once again, to have given birth in

1. On November 24, 1883, Eugène Poubelle, the Prefect of the Seine, signed a famous bylaw that obliged Parisian property owners to provide each of their tenants with a receptacle and a cover.

2. *Pot-Bouille* by Émile Zola, the second volume of the series *Les Rougons-Macquart*.

her bed and in her home. It was true that, during the first sixty years or so of the 19th century, and despite better training for its health-care workers, hospitals remained frightening places where illnesses and infections were propagated rapidly. Those institutions received only unmarried girls or the impoverished. As a subject of research for medical students, without any respect for her dignity, the new mother found herself entrusted with two or three new-borns to breast-feed, but her own baby was kept away lest she be tempted to favor it[3]...

Confined to bed, her back propped up by two thick pillows, Madeleine calmly regained her breathing and moistened her lips with an invigorating broth. Her hands felt her stomach which appeared to her desperately empty, she did not know yet that the same scene would take place again for the birth of Victoire Madeleine in 1869, Henri Joseph in 1871 and Pierre in 1872. Pierrot would be the last of "the bloody bunch" as she called her brood coarsely. Old mother Mandragore was bustling around the little body with precise gestures, making sure that the reflexes and tonicity were fine, and turning around with the little one wrapped up in her arms, she added:

"This infant is really plump and must weigh a good seven pounds!"

Madeleine Weber finally got to meet this washed, dried and swaddled nursling. The trousseau was put together with old sheets which wear-and-tear had softened into lingerie. Mother and daughter observed one another. Their slate-like stares magnetized one another and blended into one.

Suddenly, the faces of Marie-Anne and Joseph, still crumpled from sleep, appeared in the opening of the bedroom door. Dagobert preceded them and motioned to them to come over to their little sister. Their eyes, as round as saucers, were unable to remove themselves from that little crinkled thing which was swallowing every time it sucked. Dagobert and Madeleine watched, with tenderness, this starved little creature constantly moving that didn't appear satiated after that first feed. On this morning of July 12, 1866, Louise Joséphine Weber had just made her entrance into the neighborhood of Paradis.

---

3. Georges Duby, Michelle Perrot, *Histoire des femmes en Occident*—volume IV, « Le XIXe siècle », Éditions Perrin, 2002.

-II-

On July 19, 1870, France declared war on Prussia. Louise had just celebrated her fourth birthday; dancing was already an integral part of her body.

> As a young child, I had a passion for dance. When a Barbary organ passed through the alley where we lived in a very simple labourer's lodging, my mother would push me ahead of her and I would do a waltz. I came up to her belly. She began by giving ten and later twenty and up to forty cents to the musician, and sometimes I would go down into the street accompanied by the big organ repertoire. My mother could no longer get me to come back in because I was so happy.[4]

With her father Dagobert, she learned the dance step called "le chahut" (the art of lifting up one's leg) — the "chahut" was the first name for the cancan (the art of lifting up one's skirt) danced by couples at the beginning of the 19th century—and would sing the "galop" tune created by Offenbach for his comic operetta *Orphée aux Enfers* (Orpheus in the Underworld).

> This ball is original
> With its galop infernal
> Let's all give the signal
> Long live the galop infernal!
> Let's give the signal
> Friends, long live the ball
> Long live the ball.[5]

It was no longer Louise Joséphine who, perched on the table of guests at a wedding or a banquet, set the tone for the party, but the spiritual heiress of the queens who reigned over the Mabille Brothers' ball. The audience was enchanted. The little girl swayed her hips and whirled her arms and legs

---

4. Excerpt from the diary of Louise Weber, known as La Goulue, with the kind permission of Jean-Luc Pehau-Ricau, Director of Marketing and Public Relations at the Moulin Rouge.

5. Excerpt from *Orphée aux Enfers*, comic operetta by Hector Crémieux and Ludovic Halévy, music by Jacques Offenbach, created in 1858 at the théâtre des Bouffes-Parisiens, then in a second version in 1874 at the théâtre de la Gaîté.

around like a demon possessed. People were whispering in her father's ear that Céleste Mogador or Élisa Sergent, called Queen Pomaré, would not find anything to criticize in the demonstration of this young performer who was jigging about with every ounce of her energy. The little one was gifted, but it would be necessary to wait several more years until she would surpass Marguerite Badel known as Rigolboche. This very same Rigolboche who used to pull her skirts up to her waist just to expose her legs, contrary to the dancers of naturalist quadrilles who would latch on to their skirt at the chest in order to form a lace corolla.

> In 1857, it was up to the danseuse to transform the chahut into the cancan by inventing the mechanical series of leg-lifting reaching eye-level executed at a frenzied rhythm. In this choreographic system the little legs invent for themselves a subversive language, the figures, positions and steps of the cancan are founded on the suppleness of the legs[6].

The cancan was exported to the United Kingdom in 1861. Louise was not yet born, but a certain Charles Morton rebaptized it "the French cancan."

Young Mademoiselle Weber was chafing at the bit. In front of the only mirror in the house, with a sulky pout, she struck up poses and sought out the most gracious ones to impress an imaginary public. The little girl improvised a mimed dialogue. With grace and elegance, she would forget, thanks to a dance, the neighborhood of la Révolte, a place where cat burglers and other criminals rubbed shoulder, especially the Fabre brothers who terrorized her. They gave her the nickname of chickweed vendor and took a sadistic pleasure in threatening to cut off one of her fingers, the one that displayed a little ring, a gift from one of her aunts. Her nights were filled with nightmares where old beggars with their craggy faces and teeth rotting from litres of Aramon would come looking for her to rob her of her money. Her meager takings, picked up on the rue de la Goutte-d'Or thanks to selling flowers, were indispensable to keep the family going. Music was entering her body and she was singing loud enough to rupture her eardrums. Her voice liberated her fears and torments. She wanted to

6. Nadège Maruta, *L'Incroyable histoire du cancan. Rebelles et insolentes, les Parisiennes mènent la danse,* Éditions Parigramme, 2014.

silence her fears, thumb her nose at fate by screaming louder, kicking her leg higher and chasing her anguishes beyond the toll barriers. At the last note, the last dance step, she won the match, drunk with joy and gratitude in the face of so much applause. The following days, another kind of music made its appearance. The fervor surrounding the conscripts dressed in their greatcoat of blueish steel grey and their madder-coloured trousers ("not one button is missing on their gaiter!"[7]) was such that many did not doubt that the whole of France was behind them:[8]

> "It wasn't just a million men who went off to combat the Prussians but rather thirty million citizens fired up by the same patriotic inspiration," wrote Lieutenant Larbalétrier...[9]

After fifteen days of preparations, the two armies confronted one another, and the French army collapsed. The military marchpast was transformed into a debacle. In a few weeks the enemy was at the gates of Paris. The Prussians would make their entrance there on March 1, 1871... It was necessary to abandon the house while praying that it would not be vandalized or bombarded. With her round belly and rage in her heart, Madeleine moved in with her family in the 17th district of Paris, on 18 rue Gathey. The Clichy bridge, barely completed and whose foundations had been dug the year Louise was born, was destroyed in its entirety.

The siege of the capital would last five months.

The Webers would know hunger; like the besieged population, they lived on vegetables, then on roots. Meat became scarce so people ate rats, dogs and cats... Since the zoological garden could no longer afford to feed its animals, it put them up for sale. The English butcher shop Chez Roos, located at 173 boulevard Haussmann, proposed to its clients, under the name "fancy meats", dwarf zebus, Atlas stags, peacocks, Gambian geese, but also the flesh and trunks of the two elephants Castor and Pollux.

---

7. Spoken by Marshal Edmond Le Boeuf.

8. Jean-François Lecaillon, *Les Français et la guerre de 1870,* Éditions Bernard-Giovanangeli, 2004.

9. Letter from an officer published on the initiative of Captain H. Klotz.

As for Louise, she would declare, several years later, that she had eaten some lion! With nothing to do, children were entertaining themselves by watching balloons taking off whose occupants were carrier pigeons, the only links between Paris and the provinces. These mail balloons enabling Parisians to keep in touch with the rest of the country were built in the large hall of the Élysée Montmartre which was transformed into an "aerostatic workshop." On October 7, 1870, Léon Gambetta flew off from Montmartre in a balloon to join up with the provisional government of France that had withdrawn to Bordeaux... What was little Louise dreaming about when gazing a these hot-air balloons? She couldn't imagine that soon all eyes would be fixed on her, the rising star of the Élysée Montmartre...

Left to their own devices, the Weber children could run up to the fortifications to observe the Prussians through a telescope.

On January 28, 1871, at eight in the evening, the armistice was signed for twenty-one days. As soon as the announcement was made known, Parisians rushed towards the countryside.

> All these people, men and women, coming from the Neuilly bridge formed a strange procession. Everyone was burdened with bags, necessities, their pockets were bulging with things to eat...[10]

The Webers, however, like most of their fellow-citizens, were crushed by the news of the annexation by the Germans of Alsace as well as a good third of Lorraine. On February 28, 1871,[11] accompanied by two neighbors, Dagobert, a painter and decorator for one and a rubber craftsman for the other, brought to the attention of the officer at the registry office in the 17th district of Paris the birth of Henri Joseph, his fifth child. During the confusion, the parents did not know that the communal House in Clichy had moved temporarily to 38 rue Saint-Pétersbourg, within the walls... The bombings had spared the home of Madeleine and Dagobert as well as their neighbors', the Daughters of Charity, a providential place for all the inhabitants fleeing the Paris Commune, which had voted for

10. Edmond de Goncourt, *Journal*, January 1871.

11. The Paris Archives, birth certificate #479.

the separation of the Church and State, the proclamation of secularism and free education. The brood would not run towards City Hall to cry out its joy or dance on the square called “la Place de Grève” but would accompany little Joseph to his last resting place. The little angel did not survive all that noise and fury.

Dagobert picked up his Alsatian accent again and cursed his lousy life with many swear-words.

Madeleine, worn out and exhausted from all the hardships suffered, allowed her children to run off in all directions.

-III-

Louise was standing on the threshold of the Noiset laundry. The city of Clichy boasted in the 19th century thirty or so laundries. It was in one of them that Madeleine worked with her daughters, including Louise, thirteen years old.

Her impish eyes were observing the photographer hampered by his bellow-camera and bag filled with glass plates. The man was responding to an order from the owner of the laundry. Since 1876 postcard publicity was in fashion. After setting up his tripod on the opposite sidewalk, he made a sign to her, with a movement of his hand, to remain on the steps. A so-called vivid card brings in more customers than a deserted street. The adolescent's heart skipped a beat, she could feel the throbbing resonating in her whole body, her legs were shaking a bit, her face was turning crimson. Her fingers pulled at a lock of hair in her chignon piled up very high at the top of her skull, then fixed the kiss curl with lots of saliva. Émile, the son of one of the laundresses, came up to join her. Both were elbowing one another and having a quiet laugh. The young girl wiped her hands on her apron, a soft warmth burned in her stomach. Her steel blue eyes stared at the man who was bustling around the square box. With her body turned towards the lens and a sullen pout, she struck a pose in front of this artist who had just buried his head under the black veil.

“Come on now, children, give me a little smile, don't move anymore.”

Obeying the photographer's order, like statues, they strove to remain immobile. The man was pleased, the image was in the box. Although she didn't enjoy being handled like a child, Louise burst out into sonorous laughter, slapped her round and firm thighs with her hand, then went back into the laundry. Her mother was getting ready to give her a smack which she avoided skillfully and swiftly.

"My daughter has a devil in her body! Will you concentrate on your work instead of putting on airs…"

While moving the Pole, the little iron curved at both ends, into the headdresses, Louise liked to lift up her ankles one after the other and imitate dance movements. Her mother was irritated by this, but the other laundresses enjoyed it and their laughter encouraged her to defy maternal authority. Louise was typical of her era that wanted to forget the disaster at Sedan, the Commune and the Third Republic that made the cancan disappear for ten years. Parisians resumed frequenting dance halls, giving birth to a new generation of cancan dancers, both male and female. What her mother pretended not to know was that on public holidays her daughter lead the Chahut along the "fortifs,"[12] called "that black belt,"[13] because public lighting had not been granted to a territory unfrequented by the right kind of people. The police rarely appeared in this landscape without road signs, which transformed it into a refuge for a shady class of people. Louise mixed with these low-class individuals working on Haussmann's projects, with the mobsters and their operations. The atmosphere of dance halls of ill-repute where wine flowed like water drew her like a moth attracted to artificial lights. Day belonged to the hard-working little people, night was the domain of those who went for parties, pleasure, fighting, and furtive encounters with streetwalkers. Louise was stifling in the heavy vapors of the laundry. In the hot air a stench would rise from the dirty clothing that was being thrown around. Her naked arms buried in the wicker baskets would pull out quantities of shirts made yellow from filth, rags stiffened from the grease on them and socks stiff from sweat. The steam from the soapy water, the noise of the wringers, the spurts of white smoke and the whiffs of bleach made her uncomfortable and annoyed her.

12. The name given to the former fortifications in Paris where a marginal society set itself up.

13. Madeleine Leveau-Fernandez, *La Zone et les fortifs*, Éditions Le Temps des Cerises, 2006.

Only one desire made her come alive: to wear beautiful clothes and send her beater and iron flying over the dryers in the shed. The few dance steps she did while lifting up her skirts reminded her of the dinners she used to liven up with her father. The carpenter, who would boldly hasten to adjust struts and hang whole houses on cross beams, fell to his death. The Grim Reaper visited the rue de la Révolte more than enough times. The road to the cemetery had become a walking path, then life went on as usual. Madeleine moved in with Arnaud. This father-in-law brought in his salaries every fifteen days and sometimes would offer a dress to each of the Weber girls.

> He did not have my mother's ideas, he taught us catechism and the history of France.[14]

And even if he did improvisations on revolutionary songs like *Marceau, Hoche et Kléber* and *Moselle en sabot*, another kind of excitement attracted her, every evening, around the Clichy barrier. The young girl would take advantage of a few instants of freedom to run away from her mother's supervision and borrow the rustling undergarments of customers that she had to deliver to their homes. This was not her first act of disobedience because she had already spirited away satin slippers brought in by a high-wire performer who wanted them cleaned. Dressed in these shoes she celebrated her first communion! When she returned from the popular dance ball, she was treated to some resounding clouts.

> I came in late. My mother, the poor woman, slapped me around. So much so that at the end, I threatened her:
>
> - I'm going to move in with somebody, you'll see. And I'll dance all night long.
> - Miserable wretch! And your virtue…
> - My virtue? If you pass by Saint-Ouen island, provided that my virtue has been patient, you'll find it still there…[15]

---

14. Excerpt from Louise Weber's diary, *op. cit.*

15. Georges Michel, the pseudonym for Georges Dreyfus, *En confessant Mistinguett, Polaire, La Goulue, Émilienne d'Alençon, Yvette Guilbert et Mlle Otero*, Albin Michel, 1926.

The violent slap left red imprints on Louise's cheek. Despite her mottled cheek and the tears that welled up at her eyelids, she did not drop her guard, and, more insolent than ever, withstood her mother's stare. Madeleine understood that her daughter no longer belonged to her... With her shoulders stooped, her head buried in a body that had become ungainly, she gave up and went back to bed. Tomorrow would be another day, exactly like the one before.

Louise did not like fights; she was not a bad girl but if she went from one ball to another and danced until her heart was ready to give out, it was to return to her childhood, to the time when her father was still alive. Her complexion like a ripe peach and her mischievous head "adorned with golden hair" whose "heavy coil, rolled up very high resembled the crest of a helmet,"[16] had drawn the attention of a handsome gunner.

> I was thirteen years old. It was a summer night. My heart felt completely swollen [...] I said to myself: "A military man will surely bring me happiness." I remember. It was a lovely day, but there was a bit of wind, and the leaves were quivering on the poplar trees, were quivering... I was thirteen years old.[17]

-IV-

1882. Louise was a young woman of sixteen. At present she still worked as a laundress not far from the théâtre des Batignolles. The owner considered her kind and lively, and because of these two qualities she would send her on errands to her customers: middle-class ladies and a few tarts. The young woman would deliver the lovely and clean clothes to the clientele in the Europe neighborhood. Her senses were aroused, her eyes scrutinized the interiors of these wealthy apartments where the bourgeois called on the talent of decorators. The zinc sculptures had a bronze patina, the tapestries became trompe-l'oeil backgrounds and the imitation stone made it possible to realize fake sculptured decors.

16. Jean Lorrain, quoted in *Le Cirque dans l'Univers,* numéro 60 – Henry Thétard, 1958.

17. Georges Michel, *op. cit.*

The customers, whose gallant messages she would transmit, were often elderly gentlemen who gave her a few coins in exchange for perfumed love notes delivered to demi-mondaines. The adolescent became a desirable go-between.

"Everything in her was spontaneous and sincere, she was the beautiful young girl who suspected neither modesty nor constraint, whose nature, overflowing with voluptuous sap and fleshy vitality, opened up like an ingenuous and perverse flower."[18]

Often accosted during her errands, she was an easy prey for the young pimps who loitered along the boulevards. Like keen bloodhounds, they could smell in her the winner, the money pot, the bawdy girl dancing with the right foot in the gutter and the left one in the space between the bed and the wall. With haughty demeanor, she did not react to their idle solicitations. Those conversations bored her because she could not get in a word edgewise.

"She could have written an exam on slang and conquered the highest honors right off the bat."[19]

Her appetite for life and cheeky humor would build her legend. To increase her revenue she sold flowers in addition to wielding the mechanical iron and doing errands for her bourgeois clientele. Between Place Pigalle and boulevard Rochechouart, while handing out with her skillful fingers one-cent buttonhole violets to various gentlemen, she would observe the painters at the Butte who had come to shop around at the "models market." The girls who were not chosen to model remained in the vicinity to exercise other talents among the Johns whom they could pick up once night fell.

Louise was no exception: she peddled her charms, sometimes in the modest outfit of a seamstress who was displaying her work, sometimes in mourning as a heartbroken widow and even as a shop girl. She was not loath to disguise herself and between two quickies survived with a dear lady-friend in a small furnished room in the Batignolles area.

18. Octave Lebesgue, a journalist known under the pseudonym of Georges Montorgueil, *Paris dansant*, Éditions Théophile Belin, 1898.

19. Anonymous, *Grille d'Égout et La Goulue, Histoire réaliste,* Imprimatur. H. Marot, 1885.

By temperament she loved dance halls and living it up was her vocation. She was not a sex vendor nor even an ordinary prostitute; no, she was never anything else except a simple rover. To all those who wished to slip a ring on her finger, she would reply by spitting out the word "flesh." Neither God nor master.

One lucky night, her footsteps led her up to the Butte, to the top of the stairs leading to the rue Tholozé where stood the Moulin de la Galette. It began as an authentic wheat mill, a former Blute-Fin (Flour Filterer) disaffected since 1830. The descendants of the millers, whose ancestors had been miller-farmers for the Dames de Montmartre, had set up a dance hall there; a family clientele would come not only to dance but also to eat the rye bread which, according to legend, the old man Debray, the owner of the place, used to serve with a glass of wine or milk. In 1882, the house specialty was hot wine spiced with cinnamon and clove.

Louise pushed open the door painted in rose and garish green surmounted by a circle of white globes where one could read: DEBRAY BALL. At the wicket she had to pay twenty-five cents for the entrance ticket (double for the men). She waved politely and discretely to the woman in the cloakroom, even though she had neither a hat nor a purse to leave with the latter, which meant saving two cents. It was quite an achievement to reach the dance floor. Her buttoned boots scraped the earth corridor. Her eyes swept lightly over the walls covered with pastoral canvasses and garden scenes. At the end of the passageway, there was a luminous hall whose perimeter was strewn with tables and benches. A balustrade of red wood encircled the dance floor. The orchestra was on a platform. People danced only on Sundays and holidays, from three o'clock in the afternoon till eleven o'clock at night. The glassed-in warehouse, rather dark and dusty, and transformed into a ballroom, was invaded by:

> A clientele of novelty shop clerks, errand-girls, laundresses, workers from Batignolles chaperoned by their mothers, kids who escaped from the paternal dwelling after arranging a kiss-curl with salad oil and whose boyfriends were waiting for them at the corner of the Girardon dead end.[20]

20. Henri Perruchot, *La Vie de Toulouse-Lautrec*, Librairie Hachette, 1958.

On Monday nights one could add to this sane social category of working people and employees a collection of good-for-nothings, gangsters and pimps. Bellville moved over to provoke Montmartre. The dark little neighborhood streets had a dubious reputation. Gangs came to settle their quarrels, heavily armed with knives and pistols…

> In this dump where the perfumes that hung heavy in the atmosphere were not sensual and the dresses did not stick to the skin.[21]

To the sound of music where the brass dominated, the ordinary people were slumming it, wriggling, and jumping enough to make the chandeliers shake in front of the painters seated at tables. A man, dressed in a black frock coat, yellow pants and wearing a top hat, stood in front of Louise and invited her to dance. His face as though slashed by a saber blow and with a mouth devoid of teeth strove nevertheless to appear amiable.

"That will be two cents for the waltz," the cashier demanded while caressing the leather of his purse containing the dance money.

With a sly expression, Louise took a quick, hard look at the man opposite her who had just taken the money from one of the pockets of his pants. The brazen and laughing damsel was amused by his boney face and protruding chin surmounted by a large, hooked nose. She compared him mentally to a Punchinello figure. They made each other's acquaintance while dancing the *Valse des roses* (The Roses Waltz) created by Olivier Métra.

"My real name is Jules, but ever since the public proclaimed me the king of the jig, my nickname is Valentin. Why are you laughing, you nipper?"

Louise looked sideways at this beanpole who continued sending spitballs in her ear: "Dancing is my drug, my ether, my morphine and the way you wriggle leads me to believe that you have become as hooked as I am!" If Louise did not utter a word, she nodded affirmatively. Her eyes were sparkling with the first fires of pleasure. Her mind latched on to the verses of a popular song in the dance halls where there was talk about a

21. Philippe Mellot, *La Vie secrète de Montmartre*, Éditions Omnibus, 2008.

Valentin but she could not remember the words and that was enough to enervate her.

The dancer was no spring chicken: twenty-three years separated the daughter of the Clichy laundress and this son of a lawyer and brother of a notary established in Sceaux. While this tightly entwined couple whirled around without anyone being able to figure out the rhythm of their steps, bareheaded women were sliding on their slippers and the men, to feel less hot, took off their jackets, detachable collars and ties. The walkway surrounding the ballroom was occupied by a crowd of somewhat wild girls, with bare heads, and smooth-cheeked boys wearing caps or low hats with flat brims. They wore pants that were tight at the knees. This whole small crowd was moving about in little groups and elbowing one another to get a good view of the dancers. In the waltz, the two of them formed the most perfect ensemble imaginable. Louise was whirling around with a dizzying swiftness. Among the drinkers, two men, seated behind their beers, could not take their eyes off her. From her face all the way down to the tips of her feet, her body gave off perfumes of sensuality and voluptuousness. Her complexion became vivid under the influence of the festive mood. Impulsive, in the thrall of an animal-like recklessness that drew her into the rhythm, she allowed herself to be guided by her partner. The two blokes had met drinking beer together. They took a fancy to the little laundress. They bore the same surname: Charles. One was a mover, the other the future mayor of the city of Reims, the impresario and columnist at the *Gil Blas* newspaper. For the moment, Louise belonged body and soul to Valentin the Boneless One, even if he possessed the somber countenance of a battered Don Quixote. He, coming from a good family, she, barely pulled out of the gutter, did not know yet that they would dance together for nine full years without missing a single performance. This beautiful youngster, fresh and pulpy, was roaring with laughter, Valentin had just murmured in her ear: "You are still a virgin, less the waltz!" Her only answer was to hum the words of the song she recalled: "Ah! Valentin! Pour, pour it out! Ah! Valentin, don't stop pouring it out!" Then, imitating the gesture of raising her elbow to drink, Louise asked him to offer her a cup to moisten her "swallower."[22]

22. The word "l'avaloir" used in the French text is the slang expression for "throat."

-V-

Pierre-Auguste Renoir ushered Louise into his studio in Montmartre. The calmness of the place, its vast horizons, the quality of the light and also his bohemian life had drawn numerous artists to the hill. Before the eyes of the young woman exploded an enchantment of colours, a mass of marvels: completed paintings that were on the point of drying stood next to canvasses in the process of being executed. In the air floated a mixture of linseed oil, turpentine essence and cold tabaco. Since 1873, the artist's residence had been at 35 rue Saint-Georges. In 1889, he set up his family in a building surrounded by gardens called the Château des Brouillards (The Chateau of the Fogs).[23]

In the painter's den an ugly sofa had pride of place. It was covered with srag and old flowery hats used by his models. Louise got rid of her old gear in order to appear in Eve's clothing. Not in the least embarrassed, she was humming *Les Bottes de Bastien* (Bastien's Boots), a popular song composed by Eugène Imbert. Her agile fingers were whirling around her hair and quickly arranged a chignon perched at the top of her head and held in place by two combs adorned with two roses. She was putting on airs in front of the only mirror sprinkled with fly droppings. Her mischievous eyes lit up a face barely emerging from childhood. Louise was chattering on as though to better distract herself. Renoir arranged his palette. With his body leaning towards his easel, he observed his model. He was partial towards beautiful, robust girls with vermilion mouths eager to snatch kisses, with clear and laughing eyes, with rounded hips that had not yet known childbirth, with legs that were short, round and a bit muscular. Almost all the women portrayed on his canvasses were dancers at the Moulin de la Galette, florists, seamstresses or milliners who drew income from the enforced leisure time of the slow season by becoming models for several days.

> They are the living embodiments of woman whose conscious and subconscious depths he understood and which he could express better than any painter of his time, as well as their soul and all the palpitations of that soul. He put her in every surrounding and in all kinds of lightings where her

23. Anne Distel, *Renoir: « Il faut embellir »*, Éditions Gallimard, 2009.

> beauty sometimes fresh and smiling, sometimes melancholic and in pain, could blossom forth best.[24]

Louise had a crush on Pierre-Auguste. She often repeated between two sittings: "You, you paint, you will remain! I, I dance, I will be forgotten..." Their relationship remained ambiguous, oscillating between love and friendship. On Place Pigalle where he brought her, she learned to frequent "la louée," (The Rented One), a circle as sought out as it was closed, made up of models who undressed exclusively for the love of art. The rate of pay was one hundred cents per session, or ten times the salary of an ordinary worker![25]

The painter was titillated, he enjoyed Louise's naughtiness. Her vocabulary, capable of making a squad of municipal guards blush, did not bother him. A veritable nocturnal butterfly, she told Renoir that she would go from one ball to another, changing lovers like chamber maids, and would sometimes end her evenings in the arms of Andrée.[26]Renoir lit a cigarette, he contemplated the porcelain skin of this new bather whom he was willing to exhibit in 1887 in the galleries of Georges Petit, the rival of Durand-Ruel. Louise made herself comfortable on the sofa, with a multicoloured stole covering her lower abdomen. Half-reclining, with her arms raised behind her neck, she observed the painter while throwing the following words at him between her teeth: "You are not very talkative this morning, my Auguste..." The rascal pretended to slumber in the softness of the cushions. Her mother-of-pearl nostrils were quivering, her mouth like a setting for exquisite pearls with a coral frame would let out a little sigh. Behind the screen of her semi-closed eyelids passed the latest esthetic nude pictures of the photographer Achille Delmaet. These negatives where she revealed her anatomy without any shame were sold to painters lacking models and in the neighbourhood brothels... Louise changed positions. Her hands with their supple and agile fingers travelled down the length of her diaphanous neck, then on

24. Octave Mirabeau, "Renoir," *La France*, December 8, 1884.

25. Jacques Pessis, Jacques Crépineau, *Le Moulin Rouge*, Éditions de La Martinière, 2002.

26. Andrée Helleng, the future Môme Fromage (Cheese Kid) of the naturalist quadrille.

to her beautiful and firm bosom that she weighed in her hands like two ripe fruits. In the room, Renoir was content to whistle while growing ecstatic over the soft and heavy nipples as well as the pretty creases in his model's stomach.

-VI-

Going from artists' studios to Ballrooms, the little laundress from the rue de la Goutte d'Or had definitively thrown her clothes beater over the windmills on the hill of Montmartre.

Louise passed through the Grand Véfour on the arm of one of the two Charles she had met at the Moulin de la Galette. Charles Desteuque, known as the Intrepid Bottle-Emptier for having caroused too much, could now only drink Vichy water. This fifty-year-old functioned both as an impresario and editor of a column in the *Le Gil Blas* newspaper devoted to promoting ladies of doubtful virtue and strippers. As the Secretary of the Folies Bergère for which he recruited extras, he flattered himself on being instrumental in the amorous fortune of Émilienne d'Alençon…[27] Some journalists did not hesitate to describe him as a common pimp.

> The horizontals in Paris cannot assume the lying position which is their natural one if they have not been approved by the Intrepid Bottle-Emptier. This "intrepid" is thus a veritable Minotaur […]. The Bottle Emptier has been promoted by *Le Gil Blas* to the envied rank of major in the Cythera Battalion. He is the one who receives the recruits and registers them. He does not dress them. He does rather the opposite … [28]

Charlie drew her into sophisticated society. For the masked ball to which she was invited, he had made for her a pretty milkmaid costume in greyish brown cloth braided in black, with a very generously open blouse. The short skirt showed off her sculpted legs in black stockings

27. François Caradec, *Jane Avril au Moulin Rouge avec Toulouse-Lautrec*, Éditions Fayard, 2001.

28. « La Légende de l'Intrépide Vide-Bouteilles, » *Le Courrier Français*, 1888.

that vividly impressed the public.[29] Her beauty, somewhat curvy, somewhat Flemish, would have inspired Rubens the same way it had inspired Renoir. Louise was admiring her reflection in the mirrors of the little vestibule that led into the ballroom. Her insolent gaze swept over all the aroused males, "the gaze of a beautiful girl who has experienced all possible aversions." [30]

Louise mocked them: "Don't these deadbeats have any women at home?"

Far from making them shudder, the new recruit's filthy vocabulary and self-assurance excited the joyous revelers at the Royal-Meilhac.

In front of this assembly of men in formal attire, with sideburns and monocles, this muse of the dance from the wash house caused a sensation by shaking her metre and sixty centimetres while kicking her leg up into the air. Her raunchy voice threw out "youyous!" that were immediately repeated like a chorus by the conquered crowd.

> La Goulue was essentially a daughter of the people, a streetwalker. She was a very singular being. It was necessary to see her dance, even once, to have this opinion confirmed. She was not a dancer. She was something completely different. A kind of unconscious animal, caught in the lassos of sounds, of beats, of brass rhythms and who leaped, bit into the atmosphere, and then went off into skies that were no longer ours.[31]

Wriggling like an epileptic, she invented steps then unleashed herself like an untameable little animal. Leaping like a kid, the clinking of her milk jug was added to the rhythm of the cymbals and brass... Her coiffure could not resist the jolts caused by her contortions. From then on, she would dance only with her hair down. The blond bangs cut clear at the forehead near the eyelashes, the chignon rolled up in a tight lock on the nape of her neck in order not to get crushed during the dance would be seen from as far away as, in a remote past, the white plume of King Henry IV of France.

---

29. *PARIS-DISTRACTION*, « Étoiles 'fin de siècles' La Goulue, » Bibliothèque historique de la Ville de Paris, 1920.

30. Jean Lorrain, "L'Écho de Paris," reproduced by Philippe Jullian in *Monmartre*, Éditions Elsevier Sequoia, 1977.

31. Edmond Heuzé *in* Jean-Paul Crespelle, *Montmartre vivant*, Éditions Hachette, 1964.

Her success was immediate. La Goulue was launched. Champagne was flowing. She discovered caviar for the first time even though she declared to the assembled company that it was not worth a good saveloy salad! Everyone roared at her earthy temperament. This "Venus of the Underworld," the nickname given to her by the Intrepid Bottle-Emptier, arched her body, allowed herself to be inebriated by the alcohol and the breath of the hot snouts in her neck. A hand trembling with emotion offered her a top hat so that she could take a collection. In this silk hat the new lady ambassador of pleasure collected gold coins, but a few old gentlemen slid their contributions into her open blouse, in her shoes... Louise would always remember this moment with nostalgia:

> Ah! Children! What an evening... [...]. It was my first outing into chic society. But there were so many invitations afterwards...[32]

Louise became the lover of a wealthy man. Gaston Goulu Chilapane hung out near the avenue of the Bois de Boulogne and took her under his wing. Gaston's fellow-revellers only knew his nickname: Le Goulu (The Ravenous). One vowel separated his lady friend from Le Goulu. She would thus become La Goulue!

Certainly, she was always hungry, so she would carry her snack in little wicker baskets during modelling sessions. Yes, she would still sometimes guzzle what was left at the bottom of alcoholic drinks. Indeed, one should not waste. Yes, she enjoyed the games of love and agreed to some eccentric practices between consenting adults. A drawing was circulated where one could see Louise on her back in front of some slovenly-looking gentlemen for whom she had danced during a New Year's Eve party. With her outspokenness she declared: "I'll willingly handle twelve, but thirteen brings bad luck!" The thirst for life and sexual appetite of this "magnificent slut," as Jean Lorrain called her,[33] were by now self-evident, but she remained above all the lover of a bourgeois who managed to conceal her name.

---

32. Georges Michel, *op. cit.*

33. Jean Lorrain, his real name being Jean Duval, a heavy-set Norman who wanted to pass himself off as a beautiful young man, was a pale copy of Oscar Wilde. His extravagance would have no doubt embarrassed his model.

La Goulue did not need anyone to nurture her own legend.

The future queen of the quadrille savored her burgeoning glory. In front of the lens of Louis Victor Paul Bacard, she struck up a pose for a series of shots. A flute of champagne in one hand, a chicken thigh in the other, a plunging neckline, a diadem in her hair, her legs spread apart: one on the ground, the other casually resting on the arm of the seat on which she sat enthroned. At 19 years old, Louise was beginning to touch stardom.

The bourgeois' passion for her was starting to wane. For her part, La Goulue finally had enough of his sticking to her like glue.

She charmed the Marquis de Biron, with whom she shut herself up for a few days on the avenue de la Tour-Maubourg. Just to get to know each other better, she accepted his invitation to enjoy the charms of the Normandy coast. This new escapade provoked a violent dispute with Madeleine, who did not wish to see her daughter carry on like a strumpet when she should have been committing herself to her work as a laundress.

> She was levelling reproaches at me. I got angry with her. I was ready to tear the bonnet off her head. She started to cry, so I hugged her and told her not to worry. The Marquis gave her one hundred francs. All she wanted was the amount for his clothes.[34]

Madeleine understood that her daughter had found a quick way of paying her share. Certainly, Louise balked in her manner at the idea of living a life of poverty, but this attitude towards the future went against her mother's moral principles. Ravaged by sorrow, furious over having made a fool of herself in front of a bourgeois who wanted to silence her because of his rank and fortune, Madeleine went back into her home and never left her bed. Louise became an orphan six months later…

During this four-day trip, this new lover drove her around in carriages with curtains, showed her Sainte-Adresse where she took delight in eating shrimp. Under her Scottish parasol that the Marquis offered her, she got bored quickly and even the charms of Trouville could not alleviate her boredom.

---

34. Excerpt from Louise Weber's diary, *op. cit.*

> I was getting bored with my balls and my little gigolos.[35]

Charles Tazzini, the second Charly she had met at the Moulin de la Galette, popped up again like a jack-in-the-box. This big, strapping fellow of twenty-eight was endowed with a powerful, vigorous set of muscles that reassured La Goulue.

The strong body of that mover made of him a protector against any attacks, capable of defending her money and, if necessary, to lay into her. Louise fought back in her way:

> [...] I broke a litre bottle on his nose and did not return home to go to bed. The next day, he was looking for me in every corner of Montmartre.[36]

This hot-blooded Italian was nasty when drunk but his "Lolotte" (the diminutive that he would murmur to her in the horizontal position) did not bear grudges when in the vertical one: she had tattooed on her left arm "I love Charly forever."

At the dawn of her twentieth summer, La Goulue still had the dance in her flesh, still to the point of making her heart leap, but this pleasure changed into a trade through which, as a professional dancer, she would exhibit herself in front of an audience of wealthy revellers...

-VII-

Extremely sensual, in the tradition of Céleste Mogador and Rigolboche, La Goulue's first appearance as a professional dancer occurred in 1884 at the Élysée Montmartre. Built during the First Empire, this establishment located at 72 boulevard de Rochechouart offered the only dance show in Montmartre, next door to the office of Aristide Bruant, called Le Mirliton. The place was considered eccentric because relationships came and went according to the entertainment of the moment. When the Mabille and Château Rouge ballrooms disappeared, the important people in literature,

35. *Ibid.*

36. *Ibid.*

the arts and Parisian amorous pleasures frequented it, since it was considered good taste to be seen there. Women could only enter wearing hats and men had to wear top hats and be dressed elegantly. Gustave Eiffel conceived its structure.

> In front of the entrance, on the boulevard, carriage-door ushers, called beggars, watched for the arrival of the vehicles. Under the trees, a line of cabs was parked while waiting to take on couples after the show. Hanging over the roadway was an imposing glass awning with an openwork gallery and two statues standing like sentinels next to a Renaissance-like prominence.[37]

At the door, a string of glass balls formed an incandescent portico that extended an invitation to a public composed not only of merchants, workers, but also elegant people looking for a change of scenery. One had access to the ballroom through a large staircase with a balustrade. In the summer, patrons would leave the winter garden to dance under the friendly shade of the plane trees. Cascades, rocks, a suspended bridge, streams, turrets, discreet labyrinths (coming from the former Bal Mabille) arranged for couples seeking out solitude, nothing was missing in these gardens whose echoes resounded with the grisettes' joyous frolics...[38] The orchestra made up of forty musicians was directed by Dufour, succeeding Olivier Métra who had gone off to take a position at the Folies Bergère. The establishment was supported by *Le Courrier Français*, a renowned satirical weekly that catered to a semi-socialite, semi-artistic crowd, and their articles and drawings contributed to popularizing this ballroom in the elegant world.

The ballrooms that staged shows replaced the neighborhood ones. People were no longer coming to dance among themselves, they came to watch choreographic exhibits.

> Parisians went to the ball to stroll around, Parisians went there to malign their fellow-man, Parisians went there to show off, Parisians schemed

37. Francis Carco, *La Belle Époque au temps de Bruant*, Éditions Gallimard, 1954.

38. Maurice Delsol, *Paris-Cythère : étude de mœurs parisiennes*, Éditions Hachette, 1893.

> there, dirtied their white ties, treated themselves to sticks of barley sugar, played Chinese tops, talked politics, took a course in pastel drawing, ruined themselves, sweated, yawned. But Parisians no longer danced at the ball.[39]

La Goulue, future queen of the naturalist quadrille, would perform there from time to time until her reconversion as a carnival entertainer.

Even though the Élysée Montmartre enjoyed much success thanks to the arrival of new female dancers, the enthusiasm was not universal. This "low-class Élysée," according to Robert Case, did not deserve the reputation it had acquired:

> The entrance looks vulgar and pretentious. The ticket agents resemble bailiff clerks, and greasy ones at that. In the hall, the dancers kick up a thick dust. The women, not at all beautiful, slovenly, whose profession one can guess, cling to big bucks.[40]

To learn how to dance, there were two possibilities: the ball and courses to gain suppleness at the expense of many efforts. If La Goulue possessed a sense of rhythm, her instinctive way of dancing lacked method and order. Her arms and legs beat the air like the wings of a windmill, they threatened hats, her stray locks fluttered about like "crazy gossamer threads." These improvisations could not free her from technique.

Céleste Mogador, the first queen of the cancan at the Mabille ballroom, who had become the Countess de Chabrillan, introduced Louise Weber to Lucienne Beuze. The Élysée Montmartre was open only on Sundays, Tuesdays, Thursdays and Saturdays. Tuesday was the day for big partying: the ball lasted then till two a.m. On the days when it was closed, La Goulue's footsteps drew her to the dance school of Lucienne alias Grille d'Égout (Sewer Grate).

Between La Goulue and Grate there was a gripping contrast:

> A blond and a brunette; one plump and the other thin; one pretty and the other ugly, but both young, skilful and passionate about their work.[41]

39. *Ibid.*

40. Émile Guillaumin, *Albert Manceau adjudant*, Éditions Fasquelle, 1906.

41. Jane Avril, Erastène Ramiro, Denis Ramseyer, *Mes Mémoires suivis de Cours de danses fin-de-siècle*, Éditions Phébus, 2005.

The brunette had a jutting upper jaw, a receding chin and spaces between her teeth that were too big. She had two enormous teeth, two eyeteeth that emerged from a mouth full of lightheartedness, two grates over a sewer according to her lover, a polemical journalist who was both anticlerical and anti-Dreyfus, and signed his articles as Henri Rochefort, thus removing the particle from his name.

A carnal, ferocious, haughty, insolent and provocative woman, La Goulue never smiled. She was at odds with the codes of seduction that the winsome Sewer Grate embodied.

An excellent dancer, supple, lively, charming, Grate was moderate in her language. The hall in which the two women interacted was bright and smelt of cleanliness. A mirror witnessed their movements. The dance lesson began with the lifting of the skirt. For dancers who were most often laundresses or seamstresses by profession, sophistication and immaculate whiteness were proof of professional competence. André Warnod[42] evoked an undergarment dance and the importance of lifting the skirt:

> The first gesture is the one that lights up the spectator's eyes; it determines his kindness or bad humor.

This light, mischievous and witty gesture opens partially the curtain on the promise of unknown lands, of forbidden pleasures. It is a furtive apparition immediately hidden behind the thick snow of frothy lace ruffles. Both ladies pulled up their skirts till the belt. La Goulue watched her colleague who, with a kick, threw up her twelve metres of fabric that she seized with her right hand and that she did not lift any higher than her knee. She turned up her nose at so much modesty. Her eyes were staring at the white undergarments, the long petticoats decorated with lace. The black silk stockings stood out against the white background of swishing knickers. The black satin shoes, with Louis XV heels and a brooch on the instep hammered the ground and indicated steps danced on tiptoes. It was lovely. In her shrill voice Lucienne asked Louise to pick up her skirt and duplicate the exact same movement: "Have you understood me well? When you will be

42. André Warnod (1885-1960) was a French writer, art critic and designer.

able to lift your leg and pick up your skirt with a lively little kick, without leaning over… then you will really be ready for the ball!"

Without bending, in order not to displace her body's balance and under Lucienne's watchful gaze, Louis pinched the fabric on both sides, knee-high, brought it up briskly to her waist with a light twist of her back. With a sharp thrust of her right leg, the dancer had just lifted the lower lace of her white petticoat up to her hand, got hold of it between her thumb and index finger, with her arm fully stretched out. In a synchronized movement, the other hand seized the trimming of the other edge and brought up to her stomach a fistful of crimpled batiste. After several unsuccessful attempts where the accursed piece of fabric rebelled, the student managed to tame the undulating cloth with dexterity and fluidity. Louise was having a good laugh in her heart of hearts, she no longer stopped dancing, she made her dress undulate like a scarf by turns flattened, rolled up, stretched out, tracing artistic arabesques between her waist and knee. Grate pinched her nose. It was not the sour odor of sweat that bothered her but the carnal manner in which her student was taking possession of the principal patterns of the cancan. Louise was gifted, her hand had correctly gotten hold of her skirt that opened up wide with a fluttering of wings onto hoped for mysteries. Grate's undergarments only allowed glimpses of the area of naked flesh between her stocking and the bottom of her underpants, barely a few centimetres above the knee.

The dance teacher caught the gaze of her student and retorted: When one is dressed this way, one can safely lift one's leg. Women who expose their flesh really disgust me…"

La Goulue shrugged her pretty shoulders, her face remained impassible: she said yes with her head, but her body would respond negatively when, proud of her charms and brazen enough to reveal her "intimate efflorescence" through the lacy foam as she spread her legs wide apart, she would expose, above the garter, this little piece of naked skin, as the magazine *Le Gil Blas* would emphasize in 1881.

At the Élysée Montmartre would appear the first deviations from the famous naturalist quadrille, engendered by La Goulue and Grille d'Égout, quickly followed by other comrades using pseudonyms who would overturn the customary rules regarding seduction. The quadrille that they danced broke with tradition. With Pomaré and Mogador, the "queens" of the ballroom run by the Mabille brothers, the dance had become a show in itself but the ladies had not repudiated their partners.

> It is the woman who leads and no longer the gentleman: he responds to the freedom and sensibility of the danseuse with detachment, phlegm and coldness.[43]

The male soloist considered himself in this configuration like a rooster in a chicken coop! These women liberated themselves from social constraints by using comical, provocative, shocking or ironic sobriquets... Certain pseudonyms evoked the gutter (La Môme Caca [The Caca Brat] and Grille d'Égout [Sewer Grate], bistro accessories (Half-Siphon) and artillery material (The Explosive One), others inspired by plants (Églantine, Mimosa), animals (Pigeonnette, Fauvette), minerals (Topaze, Émeraude). The men did not want to be outdone. The Boneless Valentin, although incomparable when it came to performing, was imitated by a few pale ephebes: Break the Air, Quicksilver, Vol au Vent or Love Apple who simply carried on among the female dancers rather than leading the quadrille.

Grate, with her soft ankle boot in her hand, displaying her calf, her large black stockings and her wide lace knickers tight above the knee, would calm the carnal violence of La Goulue whose colourful dress contrasted with the more sober outfit of her colleague.

As a waltzer La Goulue would have remained Louise Weber, but she applied the artistic recklessness she had in her to the chahut and with her foot picked up Rigolboche's sceptre.

The seductive powers of these two so different young women earned them both very big successes. Grille raised the chahut to the level of a gavotte and looked like a bourgeois lady out for a good time. From the very first downbeats she began a number with conquering assurance and communicative verve, and when she danced, less lascivious than impertinent, she became witty and mischievous. She would put on a show that was less exciting than funny.

43. François Caradec, *op. cit.*

Between 1883 and 1889, the two dancers performed in different halls, during gala evenings where dance contests were organized like at the Galerie des Machines. While Grille d'Égout came second and Valentin took home the gold medal, La Goulue obtained first prize: a grey wool stocking with two hundred francs distributed in five-franc coins:

> The idea was original. What a change from my open-work border black silk stockings! This woolen sock could be useful to put away my twenty franc coins.[44]

The public was especially fascinated by La Goulue who, during her solo numbers, gave free rein to her exuberance, which assured her an early popularity inspired by provocation tinged with vulgarity. During the summer of 1885, standing on her left leg sheathed in black, in front of the Baron de Rothschild, she lifted her right leg by holding it by the ankle, and raising her foot up to the level of his lecherous stare, she revealed for the whole audience all the layers of her frills.[45] Four years later, she created the song at la Scala: "Frou-frou, frou-frou par son jupon la femme, Frou-frou, frou-frou de l'homme trouble l'âme" (Frou-frou, frou-frou with her petticoat woman, Frou-frou, frou-frou, arouses man's soul). The song was written and set to music by Henri Chatau, then taken up again by Juliette Méaly who would shamelessly claim it as her own.

Provocative, taking advantage of her position as an adulated dancer, she profited from her increasing glory among the aristocracy.

In her memoirs La Goulue evoked her encounter with the Baron de Rothschild:

> One day a tall gentleman approached me and said: "La Goulue! Tell me where you are going to position yourself to dance your quadrille?" I was having a go at the rifle range. I looked at him with his big red beard and continued shooting. I got him to pay forty francs that I owed for the shoot and I had him accompany me to the ball area to dance the quadrille.

44. Excerpt from the diary of Louise Weber, *op. cit.*

45. Martin Penet, *Mistinguett, la Reine du Music-Hall,* Éditions du Rocher, 1995.

> It was the Baron de Rothschild. He put three crumpled bills of one hundred francs in my hands.

At the Élysée Montmartre, La Goulue was performing in a dress embroidered with fruit, propelled by the orchestra directed by Dufour.

At the stroke of midnight, the smashing of cymbals followed by a long drumroll indicated the signal for the cancan. A formidable "Hurray!" greeted the first notes of the quadrille called "the belly dance" brilliantly led by the conductor, a fat man with a face verging on apoplexy.

> It was a pleasure to watch La Goulue in the large hall decorated in bright and happy colours, begin the quadrille conducted by Dufour with his boisterous baton. She started with the demeanor of a duchess who had stepped out of a picture by Latour, then she became lively, showed a double string of pearls while letting out fresh, young laughter. With a kick she brought up a cloud of lace petticoats. With the public's attention thus intensified, and in the pink transparency of sheer, tight batiste knickers, one could feel the fierce, ardent curiosity of the elegant club men and joyous revelers from all walks of life, who were rushing up to the front in tight rows.[46]

The spectators left their tables to rush up towards the ballroom floor and formed a circle around the dancer couples. The orchestra tore into a galop and, as though mounted on springs like mechanical toys, the girls started to stamp and prance about while lifting up their petticoats while the men were contorting themselves and at the same time stimulating their partners with their cries. La Goulue was whirling like a cyclone. Her skirts were fluttering above her chignon which stood up like an enormous thumb at the summit of her cranium. She was wiggling her bust so much that at each thrust her hard breasts were piercing through the transparent tissue of her blouse.

> She was a storm in the middle of the night, a veiled appeal and invitation to sex, a salesgirl of ruckuses, an electric battery, a triumphant victor of the dance communicating to a whole epoch the force of life within her that

46. *PARIS-DISTRACTION, op.cit.*

> she turned into a galloping halo in the arena where she floored all the men, inflicting on them the need to become for several minutes her subjects and her slaves.[47]

Under the gas lamps of the Élysée Montmartre, the queen of the ball lifted up her leg high, exposing her intimacy to the blazing eyes of the men, but especially of a new friend whose physiognomy was atypical. La Goulue addressed her most beautiful glances to him, without fearing the angry gaze of the commissioner of the morality police, Coutelas du Roché. A photographer by day, he worked at a second job at night for the morality police. This Father Modesty was a well-known personality in Montmartre. In charge of combating the indecency of these ladies, he took his responsibilities very seriously. Dressed in a black suit lined with a steel chain, carrying around his neck a collar of safety pins and a seamstress's measuring tape (the pins were to close the undergarments, the measuring tape to determine how wide the cleavages were), he made sure that the prancing girls did not transgress the boundaries of indecency when, in an unfurling of swishing lingerie, in the time it took to let out a sigh, they would bare a rectangle of flesh... He often came to keep the regular clients company, to tell them about his problems and to sip a hot wine.

> Very recently La Goulue gave me a few more white hairs. Just Imagine, she took it into her head to unbutton her knickers, in a swift gesture, at a given moment of the evening. Naturally, the circle around her became even larger, and, naturally as well, no one complained. I designated myself, as it was my duty, as the champion of outraged morality and which no one bothered defending. I drew La Goulue aside [...] "But I assure you, my little Father Modesty, that this is an accident..." she cried out. And she added: "Will you believe me, you old boor" [...] The next day, the knickers got unbuttoned again. But I was watching out, I was there. I spoke harshly, I threatened, I was forceful and never again did La Goulue try it.[48]

Seated in front of his absinth, marinating in the sound and humidity of the ballroom, a little guy listened politely to the complaints of a timorous

47. René Wisner, « La Goulue, Le Moulin Rouge, » *Volonté*, February 2, 1921.

48. *Le Gil Blas*, January 17, 1892.

old man whose task turned out to be impossible. He would have liked to answer him that he enjoyed nourishing his art with the degeneration and the blemishes imprinted on the faces of the dancers at the Élysée Montmartre ballroom, but he preferred to remain silent. In his sketchbook he drew forms, subjects. Absent-minded, still plunged in his bitter observations, Father Modesty did not show any interest in the sketch for the painting *The Quadrille of the Chair of Louis XIII at the Élysée Montmartre*. The painter was jubilant. In a few months, his work would be exhibited at the cabaret *Le Mirliton* owned by his friend Bruant. The two female dancers opposite one another lifted up a leg that they maintained at the level of the tibia while making a military salute. They were accompanied by a crouched man and all three derided Father Modesty who turned his back on them... As though to provoke Coutelas du Roché, each time she passed in front of the table situated at the edge of the dance floor, La Goulue came up and teased the gnome's snout with her twelve metres of lacey frills. What could she possibly see in him? His face had an odd ugliness about it: on his overly large head he wore a bowler hat with flat rims, his protruding eyes scrutinized the chap with an impish gaze, his lips were thick, his beard was black and shaggy. His misshapen body was dressed in a cardigan of blue ratine from which emerged a dark green scarf, half-undone, and the extremities of which were hanging around his neck. His pants in black and white checks were known by everyone in Montmartre. A little cherrywood cane in the form of a hammer arm, hanging from the back of his chair, supported him in his unsteady gait. Lautrec was overjoyed. He felt friendship for that mocking lady who made him forget Red Rosa, a streetwalker with red hair whose silhouette haunted the corridors of the Élysée Montmartre. While sketching a line in his notebook, doing charcoal drawings with a blown-out match of the curve of a neck, the undulation of a mass of hair or the contour of a hip, he continued drinking heavily. His drawings knew everything about the women's provocative gestures and the men's faces flushed with pleasure. Sometimes, he would wave a hand in his friend's direction to show her that he was having fun, too. A collective madness overcame the hall. In the air were floating odors of sweat mixed with odors of cigars. The spectators' obscene remarks answered the hammering of heels and the strident yells of gentlemen in the deafening growling of the brass. Picking up his pencil tirelessly, the man captured the positions of the cancan dancers, the new patterns linked together under the wild pom-poms of the musicians. The pirouettes, the gyrating movements were accelerating, the dancers, male and female, like marionettes whose wires had been broken, were falling to the ground in a final crash of the cymbals.

> The orchestra's rage announced the end of the quadrille; the bows rushed on the violins and the musicians' fingers bit the strings furiously; the brass instruments were bellowing; a tempest was unleashed, furious and deafening. [...] The race sped up, the bosom was heaving, panting, the arms were thrashing the air, and, in a last beat, the heel of the flying foot hit the floor again, extended itself, flashed by, slid away, pulling the leg with it and causing the pelvis to collapse, leaving a heavy bruise on the sex organ as it fell to the ground between the diabolical gap of the splits. And now, resting her elbow on her knee, lying with her chin in her hand, suddenly calmed, the dancer cast the tranquil satisfaction of her impassible smile over the excited crowd.[49]

Nothing escaped Henri de Toulouse-Lautrec. Everything attracted him. He would invite La Goulu into the calm of his studio located on rue Tourlaque where he would tirelessly work on her silhouette sketched from real life.

The trombones grew silent. The party was over. More beautiful, more insolent than ever, in her blouse matching the color of her eyes, with her neckline down to her navel, a satin ribbon tied around her neck recalling the Olympia of Manet, La Goulue, the queen of the ball and of the love vendors, joined her "P'tit Touffu," (Little Bushy One), the nickname she gave this painter born in Albi but who had come to lose himself in Paris.

Both of them had a good laugh like kids who played a trick on one another. Henri loved this girl whose acts of audacity enchanted him. To salute the public with her henceforth famous rear-end thrust, she pulled up her knickers, where, on her rear end, appeared an embroidered heart in all its glory. With a sharp gesture, she filched the notebook of sketches that

49. Berthe Bernay, *Raoul Charbonnel. La Danse. Comment on dansait, comment on danse. Technique de Mme Berthe Bernay...* Notation musicale de MM. Francis Casadesus et Jules Maugué. Illustrations de M. Valvérane, Garnier frères, 1899.

she waved like a fan. La Goulue guffawed: "When I see my ass painted by you, my P'tit Touffu, I find it very beautiful..."

-VIII-

The year 1889 was a productive one for France. After two years of construction work, the World Fair was inaugurated with great pomp by the President of the Republic, Sadi Carnot. The historical fair celebrated the centenary of the French Revolution and consecrated the Eiffel Tower, a monument three hundred metres high that would become the symbol of Paris. The *Courrier Français* printed on its first page a drawing by Ferdinand Lunel in which a dancer kicks her leg up high in front of a select public: "Greetings to the Provinces and to the World!", the caption proclaimed. Even though the cancan dancer was in the foreground, the silhouette of the Eiffel Tour remained prominent.[50] To make travel easier for the provincials, the train ticket was sold combined with entrance to the Fair. This double ticket offered a twenty-five per cent reduction on the trip with free baggage allowed up to thirty kilos. Entrance to the site was fixed at forty centimes. The ascent of the Eiffel Tower was five francs...

La Goulue and her little P'tit Touffu went off to conquer the vast reconstituted globe and took the urban railway on which travelled a Decauville train pulled by miniature steam locomotives. This world tour could be done in one or two hours without fear of being massacred or devoured by a tiger or a Pygmy! The black men sometimes aroused an unsettling curiosity in the women. On the Champ-de-Mars, Touaregs wearing blue veils over their faces, passed by bare-breasted Amazones from Dahomey. As the rue d'Alger rushed down from the Trocadero towards the Seine, it imitated the Grand Casbah in plaster and cardboard form. Sitting on richly colored cushions, visitors came to drink mint tea there while listening to Arabo-Andalusian orchestras. In the unpretentious little restaurants, La Goulue was offered samples of oriental perfumes and Lautrec became invisible, as though by magic, under the tents of Indian sacred dancers.

50. Francesco Rapazzini, *Le Moulin Rouge en folies*, Éditions Cherche Midi, 2016.

During the Fair, highnesses and princes deserted the official places and dined at the cabaret. Instead of dancing the pastourelle in the salon of the head of state, they went to see Grille d'Égout and La Goulue doing the quadrille, which was far more entertaining.[51] Interpreters were sent to La Goulue; her renown had become international!

> The interpreter introduced himself to me and said: "La Goulue, here is the gentleman who wishes to offer you a glass of champagne." He almost didn't dare approach me to speak..." [52]

At that time as well, Louise was leading a parallel life in the carnival milieu at the Fernando circus where she played the role of a Parisian lady with a colorful vocabulary in a show called, *En selle pour la revue* (In the Saddle for the Revue), the first pantomime revue produced by Alievy and Surtac.[53] The shows of Fernando were announced in the press, particularly with drawings by Henriot in the *Journal Amusant* and articles in the *Courrier Français*. On January 12, 1889, the news of the year 1888, mimed by ravishing female interpreters, unfolded before the astounded eyes of a very Parisian audience composed also of many artists like Cormon, Degas, Forain and Toulouse-Lautrec. Louise got attention not only through her language but her natural ability to exhibit her charms, to allude to the body in a manner that was tinged with sauciness and roguish provocation, and through the intoxicating joy of a knowing eroticism that explained her celebrity and her nickname, "The Princess of the calf." Richard O'Monroy[54] could not stop singing the praises of that very Parisian evening and cheered thus for anyone who wanted to listen:

---

51. Jacques Swell, *Le Figaro*, April 27, 1889.

52. Excerpt from the diary of Louise Weber, *op. cit.*

53. Pseudonymes that hid no less than four writers: Armand Lévy, Gabriel Astruc, Pierre Soulaine and Émile Hébrard (Bernard Delmont in *Le Cirque dans l'Univers*, number 52).

54. Richard de L'Isle de Falcon de Saint-Geniès, called Richard O'Monroy, short story writer and novelist in the same vein as Gyp, sketched Parisian life. *La Soirée Parisienne*, vol. 1, P. Arnould, 1890-1891.

> The first prize should go to the Parisienne personified. Ah, children, what an emotion! You would never believe it was aroused by La Goulue. La Goulue herself! With her big directoire hat, her full and firm cheeks, her sensual nose, her fleshy lips, roguish and pleasing like a drink enjoyed at a bar counter. Showing her shaply legs sculpted in the black leotard that gave us a glimpse of the edge of her thighs between the garters and the lacework of her light knickers, she dances with a plebeian charm while letting out laughter that seems like gurgles in an electrical apotheosis...

On the contrary, Jules Roques, a journalist at the *Courrier Français* wrote a diatribe against this rising star on January 13, 1889. The hack stressed the luminous idea of the director to mount a revue in the circus; he praised the physique and the charm of certain performers like Mlle Manon, a very piquant gossip (*sic*), Mlle Janvier, the prettiest lady in the troop but deplored the choice of La Goulue to represent the Parisienne:

> Yes...this demoiselle whom we have all encountered on the boulevards and in the nocturnal restaurants where she is tolerated, has been given the responsibility to represent and personify the Parisienne by dancing a chahut that would be very acceptable at the salle Favié or at the Grand-Turc. Monsieur Fernando, whose circus is frequented by a large number of families of petits bourgeois and neighborhood merchants, has not reflected on the thoughtless act he has committed. I am the first to applaud La Goulue in the places where she is tolerated, at the Moulin de la Galette, at the Élysée Montmartre or elsewhere. In those places she is in her element. When I go to these establishments, I know in advance what to expect. But what revolts me is that a director forgets the respect he owes the public to the point of authorizing a girl to exhibit herself in front of his audiences. We are just one step away from having the personnel from public brothels on the exterior boulevards parading here. [...] Monsieur Fernando will certainly understand that he, as they say, pulled a boner, which can happen to any good director; he will give this role to some other person less known and more reserved... I am convinced that the authors have done everything in their power to spare their performers the presence of this... black sheep whose enrollment, as a result of her morals, should be elsewhere rather than as a star in this show program. All decent people will agree with me; and my press colleagues will support me in my campaign

> to prevent the display on our Parisian stages, next to honorable artists, of sidewalk celebrities.[55]

It was true that the Magistrate's Court of the Seine had just judged a procurement scandal in which the two accused, answering to the names of Brizard and Ravet, were offering, for a fee, sumptuous hospitality to girls looking for easy money. Circus riders and theatre extras were the principal residents at the brothel. Among the infrequent boarders one could find the name of Louise Weber, nineteen years old at the time. When, at the hearing, La Goulue came forward to testify, the president, remarking that she had a smile on her lips, recommended that she show a less casual attitude. The Brizard and Ravet women got a thirteen-month sentence.[56] The novelist Aurélien Scholl, in his novel *Paris en caleçon* (Paris in Underpants), would conjure up the affair in these terms:

> Thirteen months in prison for having incited La Goulue to commit debauchery, that is harsh. One could more logically pursue La Goulue for incitement to sexual procurement. One is not always a minor because one is not yet 21 years old. The boulevards are overflowing with perfectly adult-like girls even though they have barely reached the age of their first communion. Apropos of this I remember a bit of dialogue exchanged between two Empire senators towards the end of 1869. One said: "I noticed you yesterday evening at the Café Anglais with the little Frisquette from the Variétés theatre."
>
> "Yes, I find her entertaining."
>
> "But she's been around for a long time, she is at least sixteen years old."
>
> "That's possible, but she is very well preserved for her age!"

The lord of the domain reigned as master of his circus.

> It is the circus of the exterior boulevards, located at the top of the rue des Martyrs, its popularity radiates from Batignolles to La Villette and Belleville. Pigalle and Montmartre are crazy about it.[57]

---

55. *Le Courrier Français*, January 13, 1889, Archives of the Montmartre Museum.

56. *Le Petit Parisien*, April 3, 1886.

57. *Le Sport*, January 14, 1888.

Louis Fernando, his two heavy cheeks lined with an ebony mustache, his white vest overlapping his tailcoat and his dainty feet disappearing in the volume of his bell-bottomed trousers,[58] was rubbing his hands. His popularity and his success were due to the public of Montmartre where he recruited his personnel. It was impossible for him to dismiss La Goulue from his show because the public was hurrying in larger numbers than ever to admire the beautiful Parisienne!

It was neither the first nor the last time that La Goulue would be the target of an angry press. In 1885, Emma Valladon, called Thérésa, directed the concert at the Alcazar. This cabaret chanteuse, immortalized by Degas in the *Chanson du chien* (The Dog's Song), had the brilliant idea of engaging La Goulue and Grille d'Égout to dance the famous quadrille for the audience. On November 7 of that same year, the two dancers were accused in court of moral embezzlement by the revue *La Vie moderne*. The popular novelist and journalist Albert Dubrujeaud quoted Émile Zola who, in a violent article published in the newspaper *La Tribune*, wielded an angry pen (*sic*):

> Against a public of paid applauders who swooned for an act of obscenity underscored by a movement of the hips. The day a woman will have the sublime idea to get down on all fours on stage and play in a naturalistic way the role of a stray bitch, on that day Paris will become sick with enthusiasm. What do you expect, we have grown up in a climate of shame, we are the bastard children of an accursed epoch. We are still only at the stage of swaying hips and bosom play. But be patient! The slope is fatal, we will roll down till the gutter if, overcome by nauseas, we do not recover...

In addition, Dubrujeaud stated that it was impossible for him to describe the lewd hip-swaying of the roguish chahut without committing a statutory offense that had judiciously foreseen the case where mere words could become an immoral act! The plea for the defense by the lawyer Léon Riotor insisted on the essentially French character of the cancan, a purely Gallic tradition.

58. Pégase à Fernando. À Propos de "Cirque" et du réalisme de Seurat en 1891. Éric Darragon, in *Revue de l'Art*, 1989, no. 86. P.44-57.

> That these demoiselles are morally upright or not has nothing to do with it. Everyone acts according to his education and cerebral faculties. They brought delight to the Élysée Montmartre, and I assure you that I enjoyed myself many times while watching them, these two sour-tempered girls, because, as far as character is concerned, they should not be touched with a bargepole. Are they sex vendors? I would come out against this [...]. In short, then, what is so dangerous for law and order about this display on stage of a typically Parisian dance that possesses a national character so to speak, and that everyone knows at least by hearsay?[59]

La Goulue and Grille d'Égout were definitively cleansed of all suspicions of immorality and continued waving their lace frills even more.

At the Élysée Montmartre a new spectator took his place next to Tolouse-Lautrec. Joseph Oller, the great arranger of urban festivities for the Third Republic, was looking for the pride of the quadrille for the opening of his cabaret. He was going to begin to swoop down on the Parisian dance market and on the beauty one as well. Quadrilles for the dance, and shows to display beauty, these were the principal attractions in 1889 in the world of the stage. His choice was made: a well-padded blond and her brunette partner, as thin as a rake, a bit uptight and with spaces between her teeth.

-IX-

Joseph Oller was born in 1839 in Terrassa, a town in Spanish Catalunya where he resided before coming to Paris at the age of two. This show-business entrepreneur, the prince of the capital's pleasures, was the creator of the Pari Mutuel, the théâtre des Nouveautés, of the Grand Rochechouart Swimming Pool, of the Nouveau Cirque, of the Montagnes Russes (The Roller Coaster). His associate Charles Zidler, his elder by nine years, took over the family butcher shop located in Saint-Cloud. Passionate about horses, he had constructed in 1877, near the Alma bridge, a hippodrome where he organized gladiator combats, cavalcades, chariot races and tournaments. It was also at this place that Gounod, Massenet and Saint-Saëns conducted

59. Albert Dubrujeaud, « La Vie moderne, » Bulletin de la société d'histoire et d'archéologie des 9e et 18e arrondissements. Le « Vieux Montmartre, » IIIe série, tome quatrième, années 1906-1910.

their compositions. One was tall and had white sideburns, the other of slight stature wore a beard streaked with silver strands... These two men, rather elderly for their time, fifty and fifty-nine years old, bought together an old Montmartre ballroom (closed for bankruptcy in 1884): la Reine Blanche (The White Queen). In that popular dance hall, it was unseemly for a woman to go alone...

After demolishing the ruin, a new hall devoted to woman was being constructed, but what architectural shape should it be given? Why not baptize it the Temple of Woman? The caricaturist Adolphe Willette, a regular participant in Montmartre's night life, was called in to give assistance, since the two protagonists of Parisian nocturnal revelries appreciated his talent as a painter. Faithful to the tradition of the Hill and its windmills, Willette proposed a windmill whose wings would rotate with two sculptures representing a miller blowing kisses to his miller wife! The paint chosen: vermillion red. The Moulin Rouge was born!

The Moulin Rouge was not only a hall where people danced, it was an amusement park with its wooden horses, a shooting gallery, and a brasserie. To reach it, visitors had to cross through a large garden where one would come to admire an elephant made of stucco, a picturesque inheritance from the World Fair, picked up on the sidewalk of the avenue Rapp. In one of the pachyderm's paws, a winding staircase led up to a little room where more confidential shows were offered, like the belly dance and the Pétomane (Fartomania), which every evening from eight to nine unleashed the mirth of the public by imitating on demand musical sound effects going from the baritone to the bass...

The immense ballroom, which was nothing more than a vast wooden shed supported by columns decorated with multicolored flags and gaslights in ball shapes, was located at the end of the garden. Against the elevated platform set up for the orchestra was erected a wall entirely covered with mirrors that reflected the dance floor and allowed debutants to be noticed by avid seekers of new thighs. On the sides were the galleries allowing the spectators to better ogle the dancers.

On the eve of the grand opening, Charles Zidler blared out for everyone to hear him: "My theatre will be neither a café, nor a cabaret, nor a brothel, but all three rolled up in one!"

Le Gil Blas of October 8, 1889 described the inauguration of the Moulin Rouge as a resounding success. Readers could see the headline on the first page: "*Ziedler for Ever!*" Never had one seen so many people and never did everyone have as much fun as at this première in the palace devoted to Woman, the most grandiose of temples of music and dance. Right at nine in the evening, there was a prestigious stream of loose ladies, and if need be, chanteuses or actresses, especially horizontal ones who frequented the promenades where one could hustle lightheartedly. The bluebloods and the upper crust of the aristocracy and finance as well as the flower of the world of the arts and literature, all took the trouble to come out. Just about everybody attracted by the 1889 Fair and the opening of the Moulin Rouge, du "Moulin Rouch" as foreigners pronounced it, rushed towards the hall on Place Blanche. These were the same revelers who, once they returned home, would construct pale imitations of Montmartre nights... The show took place on stage but also in the hall. One must imagine the collective delirium when it was time for the dance baptized "the naturalist quadrille" by some, the "realistic" one by others. It was madness worthy of Mabille, Chicart, Rigolboche, Céleste Mogador and Rose Pompon. Never had one seen an audience having so much fun. It was indescribable. It had to be experienced to be believed. When, supported by the brass, the lady dancers invaded the hall, whirling and lifting their legs to a boisterous rhythm, a shudder of happiness went through the assembled mass...

Of all the quadrilles scattered in the hall, the one involving La Goulue and Grille d'Égout was the most appreciated. "The fickle birds forgetful" of the cradle where they enjoyed their first success[60] did not deny themselves a good thing. The queen of the naturalist chahut dancers was without any doubt La Goulue, the pearl of the Moulin, the beloved daughter of the establishment. Up till 1894, although she no longer enjoyed the fragrance of the first flush of youth, La Goulue would continue kicking up her leg and rolling up her tulle undergarments till the navel. She was allowed the most erotic eccentricities by virtue of the adage: "Don't touch the Queen!"

60. Maurice Artus, L'Élysée Montmartre, Collection Le Vieux Montmartre, Société d'histoire et d'archéologie des 9e et 18e arrondissements, sommaire des 69e et 70e fascicules (3e et 4e trimestres 1910).

> Dancing to the strains of a frenzied quadrille, one sensed that she was swimming in her element; her eyes were shining, her nostrils dilating, a bacchant-like smile made her lips curl upwards. These lips had quivered shamelessly only for her "lady friend" or for her "gigolo." She could have followed any eccentric Englishman wild about her charms and have herself covered in gold. She preferred to preserve her joyous independence, to reign over her people of prostitutes and swindlers sporting sideburns, her childhood pals![61]

A few months after the inauguration, La Goulue got star billing. She performed at the Champ-de-Mars and at the Palais des Arts libéraux, accompanied by two hundred musicians, before an audience of conquered sovereigns. Certain ones enjoyed her intimate company. The Shah of Persia received her in a private dining room at the Café Anglais. Surrounded by eunuchs with red caps on their heads and accompanied by his favorite, he asked her to lift up her leg. La Goulue related the scene in the simplest of manners:

> [...] I said quite naturally on entering:
>
> - Hello! Sir, Lady.
>   I thought I would see a disguise and it was the contrary. Since there was no music, I saw the salon completely cleared. The Shah of Persia greeted me and so did the lady. He said to me:
> - You are La Goulue?
> - Yes, Sir.
> - Would you show us how you lift your leg?
>   I took my heel in my hand and made it whirl on the spot. Afterwards, I placed myself right in the middle of the salon, I did the splits and at the end I took my little foot in my hand and moved it about rather quickly, which made the Shah of Persia and his entourage laugh a lot. I had to get back to the Moulin Rouge for my numbers. I withdrew and the café manager slipped me fifty louis in banknotes. I noticed that the Shah was very cold as a personality. At the end, a goodbye smile.[62]

61. Maurice Delsol, *op. cit.*

62. Excerpt from the diary of Louise Weber, *op. cit.*

With these private evenings and the different dance contests in which she participated with brio, La Goulue was living comfortably. If all the female and male dancers were paid a minimum of one hundred and eighty francs per month, she received the sum of six hundred francs for the same period. By choice, Valentin was not remunerated. He would come to the Moulin Rouge every evening at the same time, like an employee. In her Memoirs La Goulue related that he did not arrive at nine in the evening like all the girls who were obliged to sign their name marking their presence (otherwise beware of the fine!):

> He always came in around ten p.m., at the right moment, and never missed [...] The boulevard residents would willingly offer him a drink, he would accept, he greeted them, drank, smiled, wouldn't say a word and went off. With her rather neighborhood accent, La Goulue used to say: "He is a very good man, but he's an *ilichestire*." This meant in popular French: *Il liche et se tire* (He drinks and goes off).[63]

The life of the little laundress who used to filch fine linen and slippers from her clients in order to go dancing belonged resolutely to the past. Her skirts were now made at the chaussée d'Antin in the famous lace shop *La ville de Bruxelles*. The quantity of superimposed flounces, one on top of the other and mounted on lace inserts obliged her, when she was driven in a carriage, to lift her dress up around her neck and sit right on the seat in order not to crease the whole outfit! Her wishes often caused chaos and she did not hesitate to go to court every time she felt cheated. As an example, the lawsuit against a jeweler who, according to her, did not follow to the letter—it was no exaggeration—her order of a diadem inscribed with her name as an artist. Having put down a deposit for the total, she considered herself despoiled as concerned the number of precious stones to be set in her jewel. Indeed, the "O" of "Goulue" was not decorated sufficiently and resembled a "C". In a fury, she maintained that foreigners, not knowing the French language, would not be able to recognize her. In the courthouse, dressed in an elegant buff-coloured outfit enhanced by a tea rose in her buttonhole, she expressed her displeasure to the justice of the peace

63. *Le Gil Blas*, March 7, 1907.

at the town hall of the 8th district: "Everyone must be able to read my famous nickname in the nocturnal lights..."

Using his conciliatory and paternal authority, the magistrate succeeded in bringing the two sides together.

The dancer won her claim and reaped publicity from the affair in the newspapers![64]

The Venus of the underworld administered her affairs as though they were a little business. Taking care of her body, she went every day to the thermal baths of Batignolles to take her vapor baths. She provided several little secrets on this subject in her personal diary:

> My waist was large and when I saw two centimetres more on my waistline, I would go right away for a vapor bath. I would go to the baths of Batignolles [...] It was also a pleasure. One would drink champagne after two massages with Cologne water. One would spend the afternoon doing all kinds of hygienic things. Things to do with the feet, the nails and hands. I would try out all the faucets...[65]

After these treatments, during which she was accompanied by her poodle whom she had sweat as well (*sic*), she returned home to her attractive apartment on the rue de Turin where her maid prepared her skirts, her rose or blue outfit for the dance at the Moulin Rouge.

This same little skivvy was bold enough to try on her boss's dresses while dreaming of glory and success. One night, however, when La Goulue reversed the order of her dance numbers, she arrived earlier at the Moulin Rouge. Stupefied when she recognized her employee among the secondary dancers, she did not mince words.

> I can understand your dancing the cancan, but you have a bloody nerve to use my clothes!

And right on the spot, the soubrette had to undress, give back the swishing skirts, pack up and leave...

64. *Journal des débats politiques et littéraires,* August 22, 1891, *La Lanterne,* August 23, 1891.

65. Excerpt from the diary of Louise Weber, *op. cit.*

La Goulue's eyes were sparkling with contentment. Charles Zidler offered her one thousand francs to mount a float representing the Moulin Rouge during the famous carnival in Nice. Every year this celebration drew a constantly larger mass of people to its very spectacular parades and its famous battle of the flowers.

Paris was abandoning itself to the joie de vivre and represented for the whole world the prosperity of the times. The seat of the International Institute of Pleasure and its delegation would move, at the first sign of frost, to the Côte d'Azur.

> Voluptuous nights for noctambulists, with their duel at dawn and their establishments boasting easy or half-naked women, where any kind of malicious gossip was in good taste.[66]

Attractively attired in a salmon-colored dress embroidered with fleurs-de-lys right on the satin, the queen of the Moulin Rouge drew all the eyes and compliments. She quarrelled with Fauvette, "a dancer friend" who accompanied her (but at her expense: "[…] I had dressed her in a pretty little suit") and who ran off with all her clothes after meeting a pimp at the casino. But she made the acquaintance on the chemin des Anges (the future Promenade des Anglais) of a certain Marguerite, winner of the Spa Beauty Contest with whom she would finish the season…

> She was a little doll of a woman, she was very blond, had almond-shaped blue eyes, a waist of forty-five centimetres and she was from Montmartre![67]

When she returned to Paris, she resumed her mischief and, as a perfect mistress of ceremonies of the quadrille, allowed herself the greatest liberties among the bourgeois who had come to applaud her.

> With an alert little kick at a spectator's hat, she removed it from his head, then did the splits, with her chest straight up, her thin waist in a blouse

66. Marie-Hélène Carbonel, Javier Figuero, *La Véritable biographie de la Belle Otero et de la Belle Époque* (description d'Alexis Tolstoï) Éditions Fayard, 2003.

67. Excerpt from the diary of Louise Weber, *op. cit.*

> of sky-blue satin and a skirt of black satin arranged in the form of an umbrella that spread out over five metres wide.[68]

It was in that position that she called out to the future king of England whose mistress she would become. They met for the first time when he made a private trip to Paris. He reserved a table in front of the stage to discover the quadrille whose reputation had crossed the Channel.

> In the generalized excitement, La Goulue descended the staircase slowly. Jane Avril, an ethereal presence, was standing opposite the sensual Goulue. To the left of the orchestra, Grille d'Égout was facing Rayon d'Or (Ray of Gold). In a flight of stunningly white underskirts, La Goulue, jumping, smiling, light-footed during the first measures, had rushed to the centre of the rectangle reserved for the cancan. Holding her head high, with her crimson lips wide open, that showed the brilliant enamel of her cruel little teeth, La Goulue was drunk with dance and music, unleashed. La Goulue gave the impression of soaring and then, landing in a flood of flounces and gold, she ended by doing the splits at the feet of the conductor.[69]

All the while she was shaking her underwear in a metronome-like movement, she shouted out to the future king of England: "Hey, Wales, you pay for the champagne or get your mother to do it!" A murmur swept over the hall. They were within a hair's breadth of a diplomatic incident. Oller's face turned livid. As for Zidler, the handkerchief with which he was moping his brow did not resist being torn in half. In a fraction of a second, with a simple snapping of the fingers, the situation was reversed in favor of the Moulin Rouge. The Prince quickly acquiesced to the dancer's request. The orchestra started to play the British anthem and the show could go on.

"Doudou," as our La Goulue nicknamed him in their intimacy, was a bon vivant with frog-like eyes and a belly that protruded under clothing lined with silk. An idle man, only pleasures kept him going. He liked merry, sassy, beautiful women whom he would invite to his table at Maxim's. In this Mecca of encounters, among the mahogany panels and

68. Yvette Guilbert, *La Chanson de ma vie*, Éditions Grasset, 1995.

69. Edmond Heuzé, « Du Moulin Rouge à l'Institut, » *in Paris-Comoedia*, 1953.

mirrors that reflected desires and under the filtered light of gas lamps the Englishman and La Goulue discovered one another in every sense of the term. Gypsies, in red dolmans with black stripes, made their instruments weep. On the butterfly-shaped sofa La Goulue once again got her wings burnt in the flames of love. As for Doudou, he overlooked her whims and forgave her her pranks. He had found his Loulou, as Yvette Guilbert wrote in her Memoirs:

> She was pretty and brazenly witty to contemplate, blond, with bangs cut at the forehead and landing right at the eyelashes. Her chignon like a helmet at the top of her head began as a lock strongly twisted at the nape in order not to fall during the dances. From her temples the classic sideburns descended in little ringlets on her ears, and from Paris to New York and passing through the hovels of White Chapel in London, all the girls of the era wanted this same coiffure and the same color of ribbon tied around their necks.[70]

The same chignon that Doudou hastened to undo…

Charlot, the mover, showed annoyance towards his Lolotte. His male instinct guessed that she was eluding his grasp. The gold set aside in rolls slid between the fingers of the winner. Valentin, her partner in the quadrille, suggested to her that she think of her future and invest her savings. In her Memoirs, La Goulue evoked her wealth:

> I adored Valentin as a dance partner and very often, I would give him my money to safeguard. When I began my career, he was the one who gave me the idea to buy City of Paris bonds and put them in the Bank of France. Valentin was a very honest guy. He always returned the money, without ever touching it, that I had given him to safeguard. At twenty-six years old, my fortune was made.[71]

Henceforth, La Goulue rode around, for the pleasure of it, in a phaeton pulled by a cute little seven-year-old mare that moved at a fast trot, and divided

70. Yvette Guilbert, *op. cit.*

71. Excerpt from the diary of Louise Weber, *op. cit.*

her free time between several private mansions of which one was called la Païva, on the avenue des Champs-Élysées. She also invested in real estate by buying for herself, in the heart of the old village, on rue Norvins, a little house adjoining the bishop's palace. Valentin unsparingly gave her advice on gardening. With a generous heart, she offered flowers and fruits to the neighboring presbytery. Charlot saw red, became violent. La Goulue retaliated, became impatient and no longer forgave either the blows or the aggressiveness of her procurer. Her nerves were raw. She had just buried her mother:

> I took care of my sick mother because she loved only me. To care for her I paid her rent and the doctor. I dedicated a dance to her nurse because she would dress my mother before she died. She asked to be taken to Lariboisière hospital where she remained for fifteen day and where she died. It was I who arranged the funeral for my mother, and I had a bier made for her of oak and gave her a sixth-class burial. The Boneless Valentin was with me, Charlot the mover and my family, two uncles and my sister. That evening, Charlot got drunk and was picking fights with me [...] and I did not return home to sleep. He found me at Marie Grande Gueule's place (Marie Big-Mouth); he wanted to hit me again. It was my friend Marie who calmed him down...[72]

This "flesh meant for pleasure," as Jane Avril would nickname her several years later, was growing tired of that lover's manners which left a blot on her new décor. Cunningly, she offered him a deal: he could stay with her but as a servant. He swapped his getup for a livery with metal buttons. When La Goulue returned home alone, after the performance, Charles became her lover again for a few hours. This lull, however, did not last long. The servant was not a lender. Overcome by a new fit of anger, he could no longer dominate his nerves and took it out violently on his boss. The police was called in and if he pretended to remove himself, he started up again the next day by breaking into her home and destroying everything in his path. In settlement, he also took off with several pieces of furniture that had resisted his anger and pocketed a silver watch and a brooch

72. *Ibid.*

adorned with diamonds. The affair came up again on the front page of the *Gazette des Tribunaux* on December 25, 1886. La Goulue, asked to appear as a witness, was mocked by the press despite the blow she had received from Tazzini. She was not a simple witness but a "witness generating sensations"; she was not a Parisienne but "Fraülein Weber who smelled of sauerkraut and headcheese salad so dear to the Beer Maidens on the other side of the Rhine." Louise was described as a "choreographic dancer in space" and her lover was designated as a mere pimp. He beat her but one reaped what one sowed…

"There was the man in the hot seat. Twenty-eight years old, a strong build, a superb jaw-lined black beard; and it was in a sad mode that this Italian as strong as a Turk and as brutal as a German"[73] related, in his way, at the witness stand, the final episode of his love affair with his Lolotte.

> In the recent past I was a kind of servant for her (La Goulue). I did the housework and the cooking. Fifteen days ago her young sister came to live with her. Louise would give me money to shop at the market but I never made a bit out of the shopping money. I told her exactly what I spent. […] It was Victorine who got me into trouble with my mistress. Louise hit me often and bit me. As for me, I never hit her. We had a discussion but not more serious than usual. When on returning at night she found me lying in her bed, she went to get the police and I did not offer any resistance. The next day, I drank more than usual because of the sorrow I was feeling. I admit that I broke down the door not by kicking it but with one fist blow…[74]

The lawyer for Tazzini, Master Pommier, maintained that the offence of forcible entry could not be held against his client. Indeed, a servant's only domicile is that of his master and by forcing the door, Tazzini was coming back home. This house employee, however, was not an ordinary servant, he did not receive any wages, he was a servant attached to a person, added the president Toutée even though he wondered, in his heart of hearts, if there was anything still left to violate in La Goulue! But before knowing

73. *Le Gil Blas,* December 26, 1886.

74. *Ibid.*

his employer, the handsome Charles had already been condemned for violence and rebellion. The court was going to take into consideration the previous history of the accused and his means of existence by inflicting on him a month in jail without remission.

Unable to get rid of the tattoo on her left arm "I love Charlot forever," she replaced the first name of her former lover with a flower and concealed everything under accessories when she had to appear dressed.

> I thought I had better erase his name because it did not look very chic when I was dressed up for the ball. I was obliged to wear white gloves and during all the parties to which I was invited, no one ever noticed my tattoo.[75]

-X-

La Goulue denounced in her way the domestication of women. She shoved aside certain codes by arriving at the Moulin Rouge holding a billy goat on a leash and thus bypassing the rule that forbade the weaker sex from entering a public place without being accompanied by a male! Her little dog collar tied around her neck, her famous "rear end thrusts," her chignon piled up high at the summit of her cranium like a Phrygian bonnet, expressed her liberation from the moral principles of her time, and underscored her art of provocation. As for her dearest female friend, that was taboo. Lesbos watched over her love life with jealous zeal. All the girls, who had become blasé early as concerned the pleasures of love, were ferociously jealous among themselves. La Goulue, overcome with modesty, was evasive about the nature of her relationship with La Môme Fromage (The Cheese Kid), an apprentice at a fashion house by day and who would join her on certain evenings in the quadrille and in her bed.

> La Môme Fromage was a basset hound turned into a woman, with short legs, an elongated chest, tubby, looking like a skivvy [...] The little dancer who resembled a dishwasher rose up and yelled: "What, Louise, you deny that you love me? Yet you aren't bored when you entice me!"[76]

75. Excerpt from the diary of Louise Weber, *op. cit.*

76. Yvette Guilbert, *op. cit.*

For six years, La Goulue carried on as the veritable mistress of the place. She reigned over the world of the Moulin's dancers and would not tolerate any show of disrespect. When she was in a bad mood, those who knew her would hug the walls while looking at the ground.

> A nasty piece of work and a vixen, one did not dare, on certain evenings, speak to her. At those moments her eyes would wrinkle, their metallic hardness would increase, and the circumflex accent of her mouth hardened as it moved up towards her nose with its thin nostrils.[77]

By clawing, kicking and biting, she defended her interests outside of the Moulin Rouge. Within the establishment, she would have been thrown out by the management, and picked off the street by the police. After the performance, she would give rendezvous to those women who were picking quarrels with her on the Caulaincourt bridge overlooking the Montmartre cemetery. That was a place where no one ever ventured, where she knew that the only ones she would bother would be the dead!

In her Memoirs, Jane Avril wrote that a poor girl named Aïcha, bawled out by La Goulue who habitually mistreated the debutants or new arrivals, stood up to the latter one evening.

> She (La Goulue) loved a good fight. [...] A rendezvous was set up on the Caulaincourt bridge at one o'clock in the morning to settle the disagreement. I was not there but the event was related to me the next day. The two women fought it out in the middle of a circle of underworld men (as they are called today) and spectators interested in events of this kind, and who intervened just in time to prevent poor La Goulue from being hurtled by her robust adversary from the top of the bridge down into the Montmartre cemetery.[78]

Edmond Heuzé, whom the participants in the naturalist quadrille baptized "le Môme Cocotte" (The Tart Kid), related that Lautrec liked to get the two women going until he could follow them into the gutter:

---

77. Gustave Coquiot, *Des peintres maudits*, Éditions Delpeuch éditeur, 1924.

78. Jane Avril, *Mes Mémoires*, Éditions Phébus, 2005, p. 40.

I consider him to be an extremely cruel man. He took pleasure in exciting Aïcha, a black model, and La Goulue until they would fight. When they were rolling in the gutter, he would separate them by hitting them with his cane.[79]

Zidler kept an eye open for problems and his wallet with absolute rigor. La Goulue got really bawled out when news of the dust-up leaked out. The director watched over the state of his company. A black eye even on a made-up face or unjustified absences were severely reprimanded. When the dancers filed past him before going on stage he never failed to make a remark: "Paulette, don't make eyes at the people in the peanut gallery! Gaby, don't laugh! Louise, don't drop your panties!"[80]

Behind his severe Bogeyman demeanor, Charles Zidler possessed a generous heart. Every Sunday, after the show, he would organize a dinner during which he would serve soup to his dancers and other courtesans.

-XI-

From the time the Moulin Rouge opened, Toulouse-Lautrec had his seat at the bar. Perched on a stool, he ordered his green fairy, then wine and champagne for himself and all the girls of the quadrille. All through the evening, he piled up glasses and sketches depicting the artists, the audience, his acquaintances and friends as well as strangers. As soon as ten p.m. arrived, he began shouting his favorite phrase: "Life is beautiful, here comes the quadrille." That was the moment that La Goulue and her favorite partner, Valentin the Lithe One, chose to come on stage. From their first encounter at the Moulin de la Galette, the rubber man proclaimed as "King of the Jig" was La Goulue's exclusive partner:

If, by chance, I ferreted him out in a corner of the ballroom with a chambermaid, I dealt his top hat a few blows; he was terrified of me [...]. And yet, he was only my dancer. When he danced with someone else and noticed me, he left her immediately. He did not finish his dance and was so

79. Jean-Pierre Crespelle, *Montmartre vivant, op. cit.*

80. Jacques Pessis, Jacques Crépineau, *op. cit.*

> happy when he would see me running after him. I would call out to him at the Moulin, so he would answer and come over quickly to me and would hold my hand to prevent me from breaking his hat and he would laugh like a good boy. It was true that I bought him his hats for one franc on the rue du Temple; because he needed one every evening...[81]

Chéret, the Watteau of the gutter as Manet nicknamed him, designed the first poster revealing in sprightly colors a woman in a tutu mounted on the back of a donkey. "The poster was magical but did not announce any magical extravaganza."[82]

On the new billboard for the 1891 season, designed by Toulouse-Lautrec, La Goulue was hoisted to the rank of ambassador of the Parisian cabaret, a veritable sanctuary for the chahut.[83] In profile, one recognized her chignon perched at the top of her cranium, dressed in her red blouse with white polka dots. She was performing the dance figure called the guitar, her legs sheathed in black stood out against a white gauze that evoked her undergarments. In front of her, like a Chinese shadow, Valentin set his grey and stretched out silhouette beside the curves and blondness of the Alsatian lady. Toulouse-Lautrec who grew shorter when he stood up, as Tristan Bernard liked to say mockingly, produced the work commissioned by the owners of the Moulin Rouge.

The billboard packed a wallop on the walls of the capital and quickly eclipsed Chéret's. On December 26, 1891, the painter wrote to his mother:

> The newspapers have been particularly kind towards your offspring. I am sending you a clipping, A real bit of honey steeped in incense. My poster has achieved a triumph despite a few errors made by the printer that have spoiled my production a bit.

Barely dry, *Moulin Rouge-La Goulue* was bought by Zidler and Oller of the Parisian night, who hung it up in the lobby decked out in purple,

81. Excerpt from the diary of Louise Weber, *op. cit.*

82. Daniel Halévy quoted in Louis Chevalier, *Montmartre du plaisir et du crime*, Éditions Robert Laffont, 1980.

83. Nadège Maruta, *op. cit.*

on the right-hand side, over the bar. It was opposite the horsewoman of the Fernando circus, acquired in 1888, at the Twentieth Salon in Brussels. The resemblance between the horsewoman and La Goulue was disquieting, given that our dancer also put on a notable performance in that circus (See page 48).

The lives of Toulouse-Lautrec and La Goulue were intimately linked. In 1893, the year when La Goulue opened the Olympia—a music hall with two thousand seats that succeeded the Montagnes Russes, easily inflammable because of its wooden structure—*Le Figaro Illustré* conferred on him the title of "La Goulue's official painter," which flattered him more than the recognition of his peers. The whole world was going to discover this woman whose outrageous antics captivated it, and who would continue, thanks to his works, to haunt people's minds. Lautrec turned her into a legend. On contemplating his muse, he declared that "there was in her a faith that no one else possessed, smiling at times, at times timid, bold or feline, as supple as a glove." Echoing him, here was La Goulue response to her P'tit Touffu:

> Toulouse-Lautrec was a really nice guy. He was rich but did not act like other men. He enhanced my stature.

The painter was one of the rare artists to perceive a savage beauty in the chahut of the public balls, an intoxication that he wished to share. His muse was not fooled by the bourgeois morality that unofficially delighted in the display of flesh but officially was critical of it. We do not know how many drawings and paintings she inspired the artist to create: a hundred or so of his works, judged immoral by Lautrec's mother, were apparently burned at the painter's family property after his death.

As soon as the year 1894 was over, Toulouse-Lautrec and his muse would take roads going in new directions. At twenty-eight, La Goulue was a tired woman, worn out by excesses. When she did not dance, she appeared the way the paintings of her P'tit Touffu wanted to depict her for us, as in *La Goulue entrant au Moulin Rouge* (La Goulue Entering the Moulin Rouge).

> With her hair dishevelled, her make up a mess, her gaze vacant as though dazed under her coiffure like a pyramid-shaped cake, her open blouse plunging downward to show her misshapen breasts.[84]

Lautrec painted *Au Moulin Rouge* (At The Moulin Rouge). No cancan. Around a table he portrayed Édouard Dujardin, a dandy symbolist poet, the dancer Macarona, the photographer Paul Sescau, Maurice Guibert, a champagne representative, and from behind Jane Avril. Behind them, on the right, La Goulue, also viewed from behind, who was redoing her hair under the enamoured gaze of la Môme Fromage while Toulouse-Lautrec appeared in the company of his cousin Tapié de Celeyran.

This canvas could be considered as a farewell gift of the artist to the ballroom on Place Blanche. It was the end of a story, of an epoch…[85] The painter announced that he was going to "set up his tent at the brothel" and returned to his second home on the rue des Moulins…

As for La Goulue, flesh was beginning to triumph over movement, she decided to turn the page by transposing her art onto the street…

84. Pierre Cabanne, *Toulouse-Lautrec,* Éditions Terrail, 2003.

85. Francesco Rapazzini, *op. cit.*

ENTRACTE

Like a robber, night breaks into my office. The two arms of the clock do the splits to indicate six in the evening. I look through the window at the almost deserted rue Lamartine. The luminous sign of *La Chope Cadet*, our favorite bistro, lights up the angle of the rue Rochechouart. The snow, replaced by a freezing drizzle, transforms the sidewalks into a veritable skating rink. The rare passersby do their utmost, through gymnastic movements bordering on contortions, to avoid breaking their bones. A Vivastella Renaut vehicle driven by a chauffeur stops in front of the door of the newspaper building. Pierrot, whose shapeless overcoat I recognize, with its pockets crammed to the bursting point with newspapers and other show business revues, rushes into the lobby. Pierrot runs up the six floors leading to my office in record time. The pallid light shines on his face flushed from the effort. Without bothering to remove his coat, he lets himself fall into a chair. I observe him surreptitiously. He looks like an elf with his little tuft of red hair hoisted at the top of his cranium. I forget to laugh at it and make fun of it as I know how to do with a few well chosen words.

"I have just gotten back from the rue des Entrepôts. Rétoré has affixed on the trailer door a rudimentary collection box and a small poster with the inscription: 'Care of everyone. This is for a wreath for La Goulue.' Our Louise was beautiful. On her death bed she recovered her doll-like face..."

Henceforth I will have to get used to hearing about Louise in the past tense. I light up a cigarette while looking at the ashtray that is overflowing with butts. Given this excess of tobacco, it would take very little for me to salve my conscience by starting to hum the song "Du gris" (Some Grey) by Fréhel:

"Tobacco is the balm for suffering.

When one smokes the burden is less heavy…"

Louise's last words continue rotating in my head like a scratched disc: "Tell them that I was a good girl."

With a nod of my head I show him the sheets of paper under my notebook and hand them to him. Pierrot plays with his glasses and begins to read out loud my last lines while making a few comments.

"As for La Goulue, since the flesh was beginning to triumph over movement, she decided to turn the page by transposing her art onto the street…"

A smile lights up his eyes. The formula seems to please Pierre and he answers me emphatically:

"A beautiful tribute to Loulou, Son. Antiquity honored their dancers by raising tombs for them: 'Here lies Septentrion the child who danced seven years and knew how to bring pleasure.' You do better than that, you are going to engrave in marble the history of our Louise…" Pierrot takes out from his innumerable pockets a wooden pencil. In a rapid and precise handwriting he underlines and annotates a few paragraphs.

I remain quiet because he is the boss. I think of our queen in the arena, of that animal tamer in that cage of wild cats and of her ruin as well… "Reine-Ruine" (Queen-Ruin). Sometimes one vowel is enough to modify a destiny. Only the staccato of the typewriter disturbs the silence of the room, and Louise's last words appear even more biting.

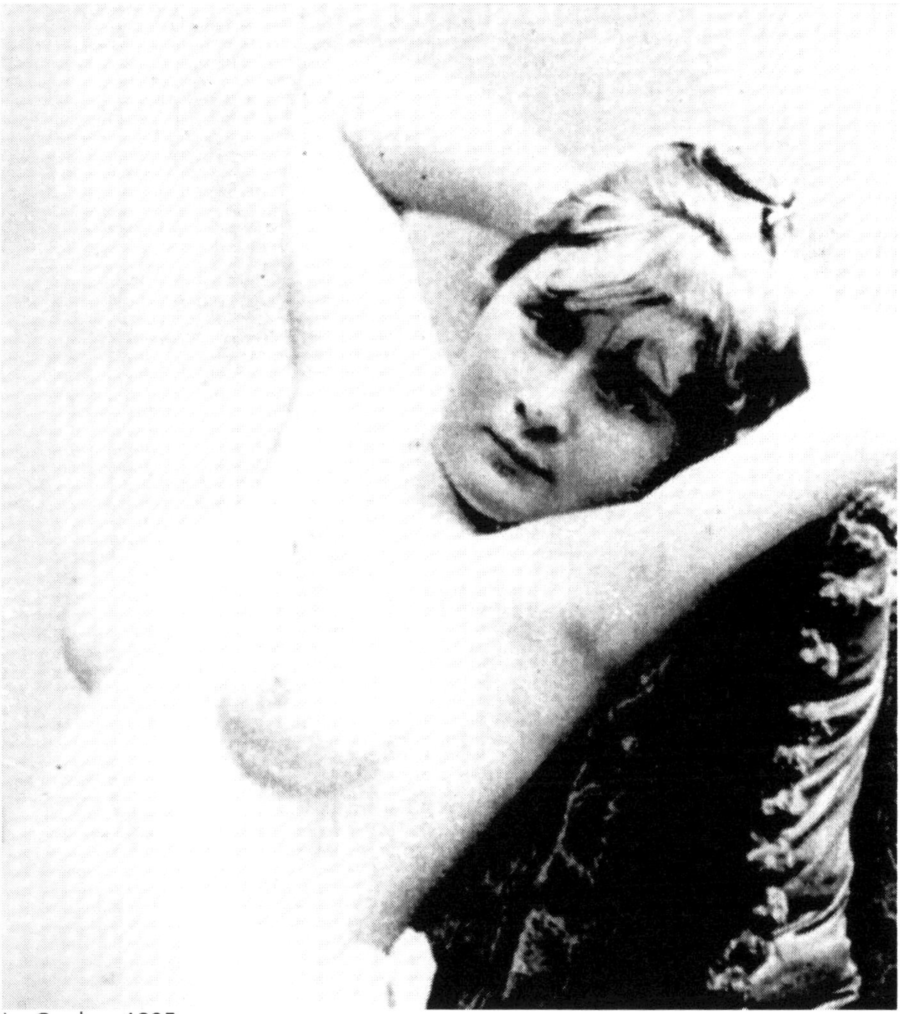

La Goulue, 1885

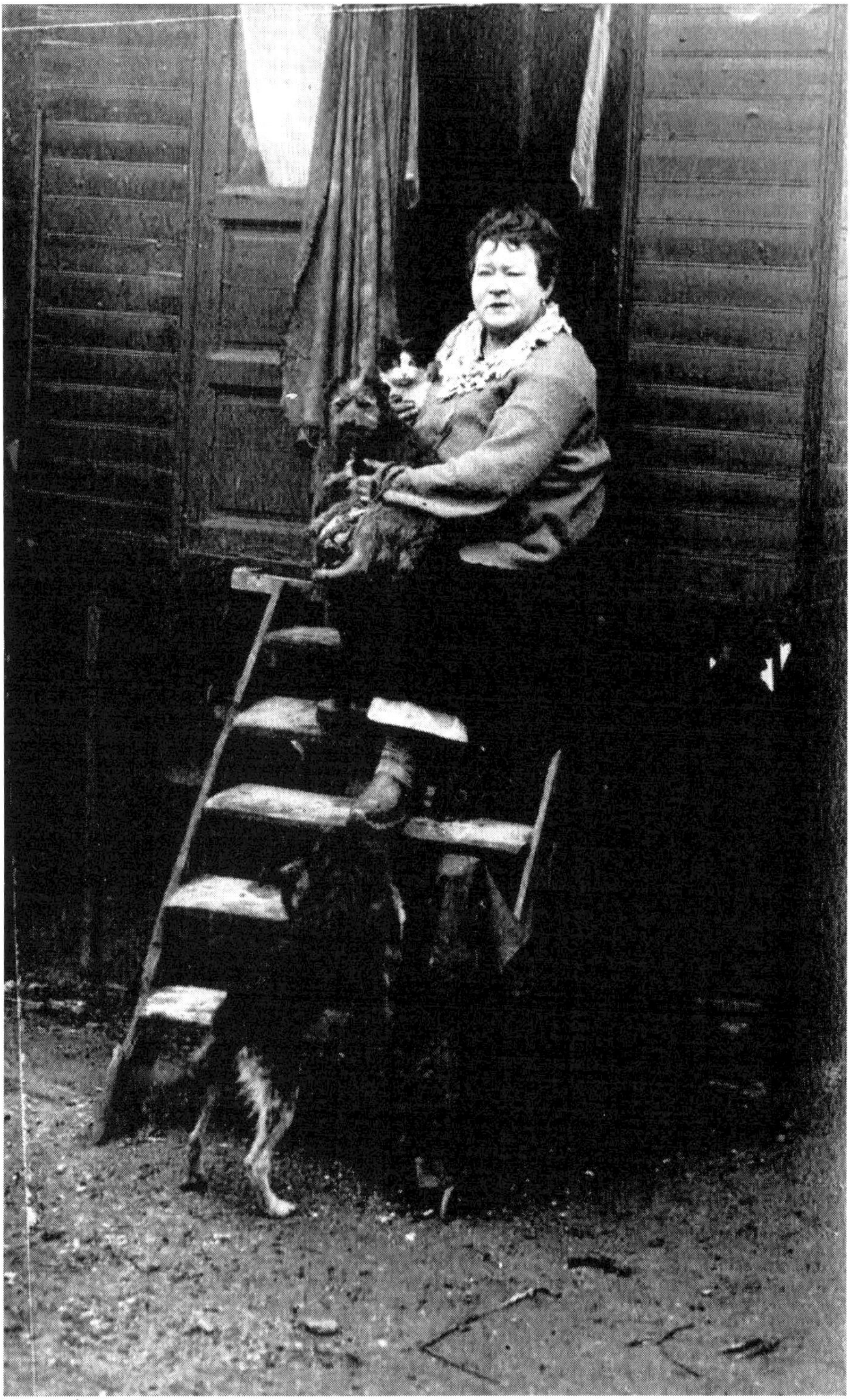

La Goulue, 1920s

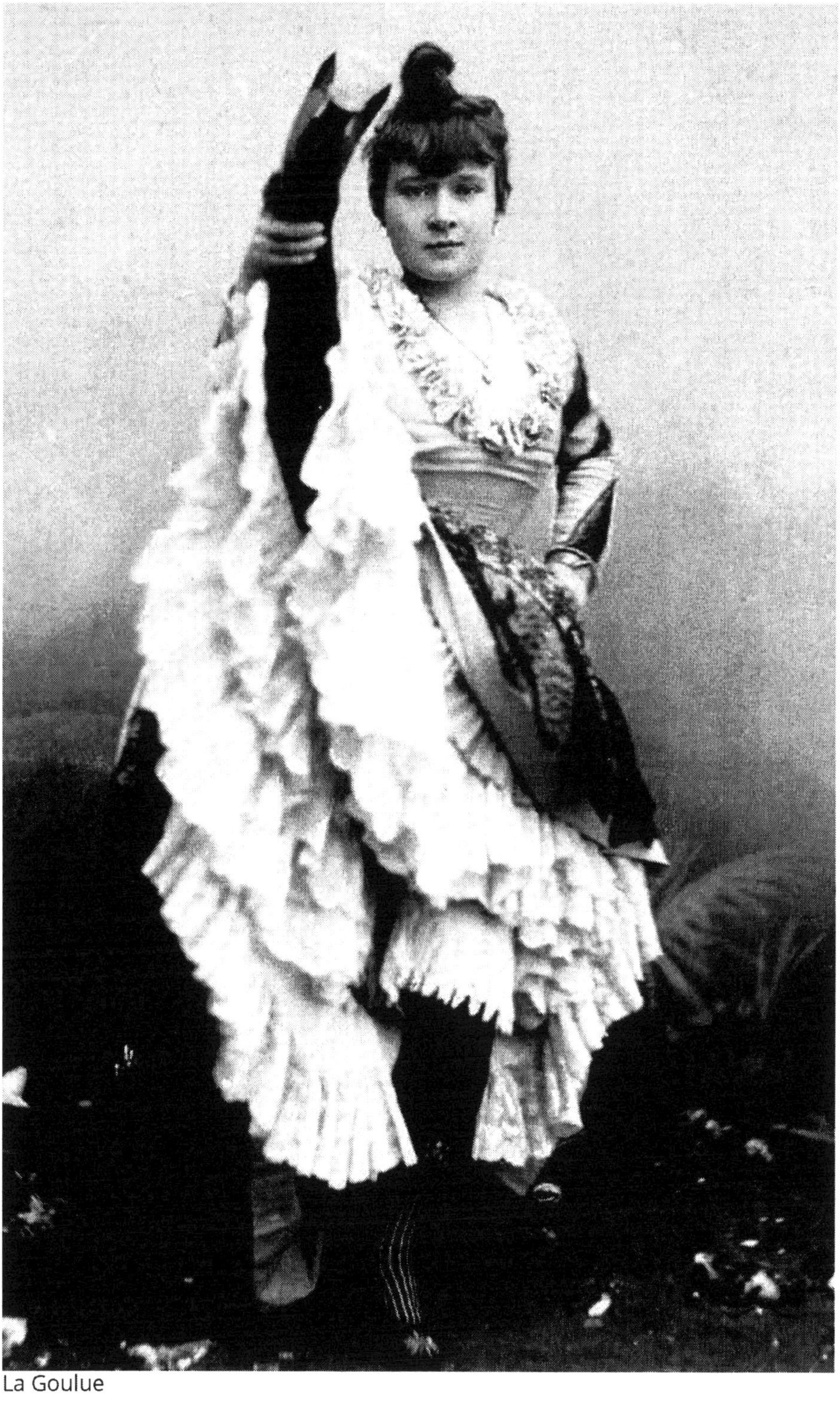

La Goulue

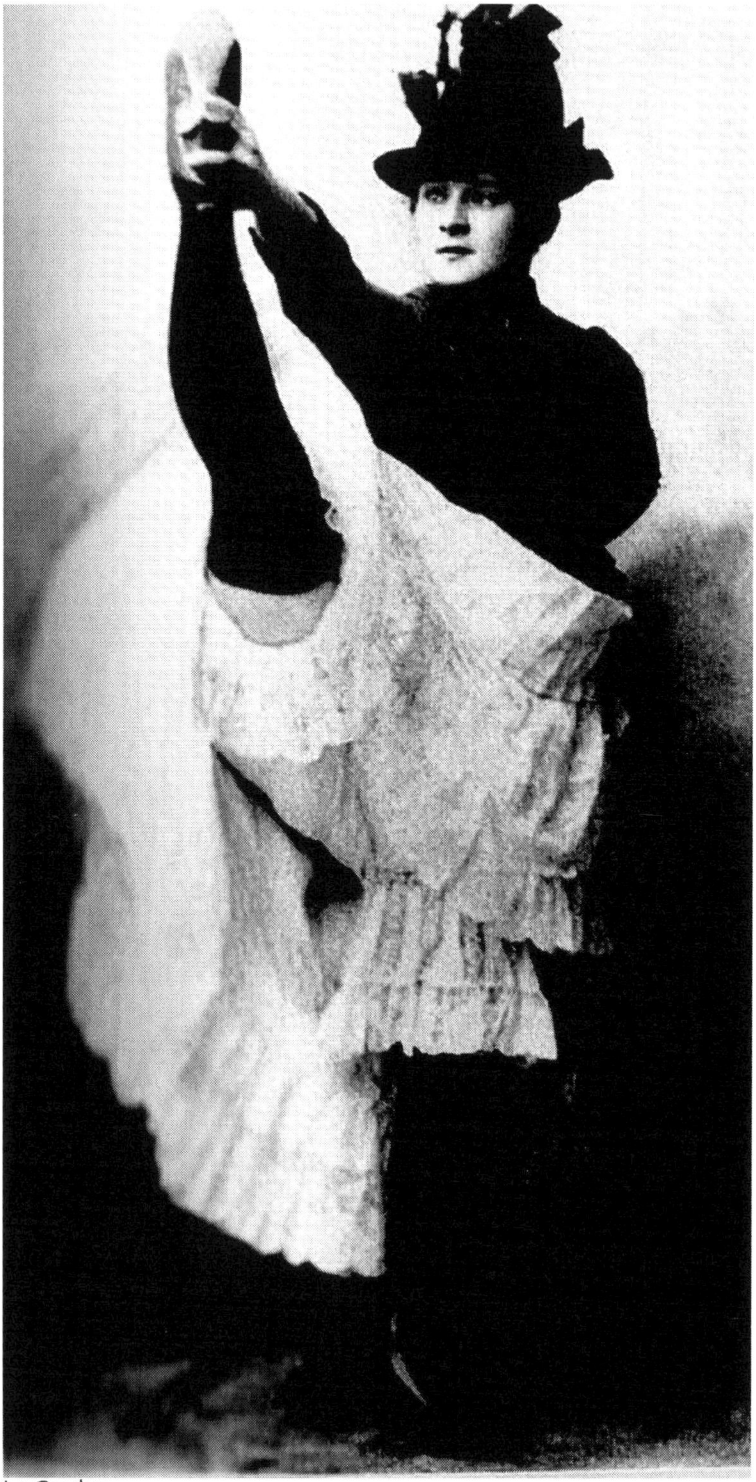

La Goulue

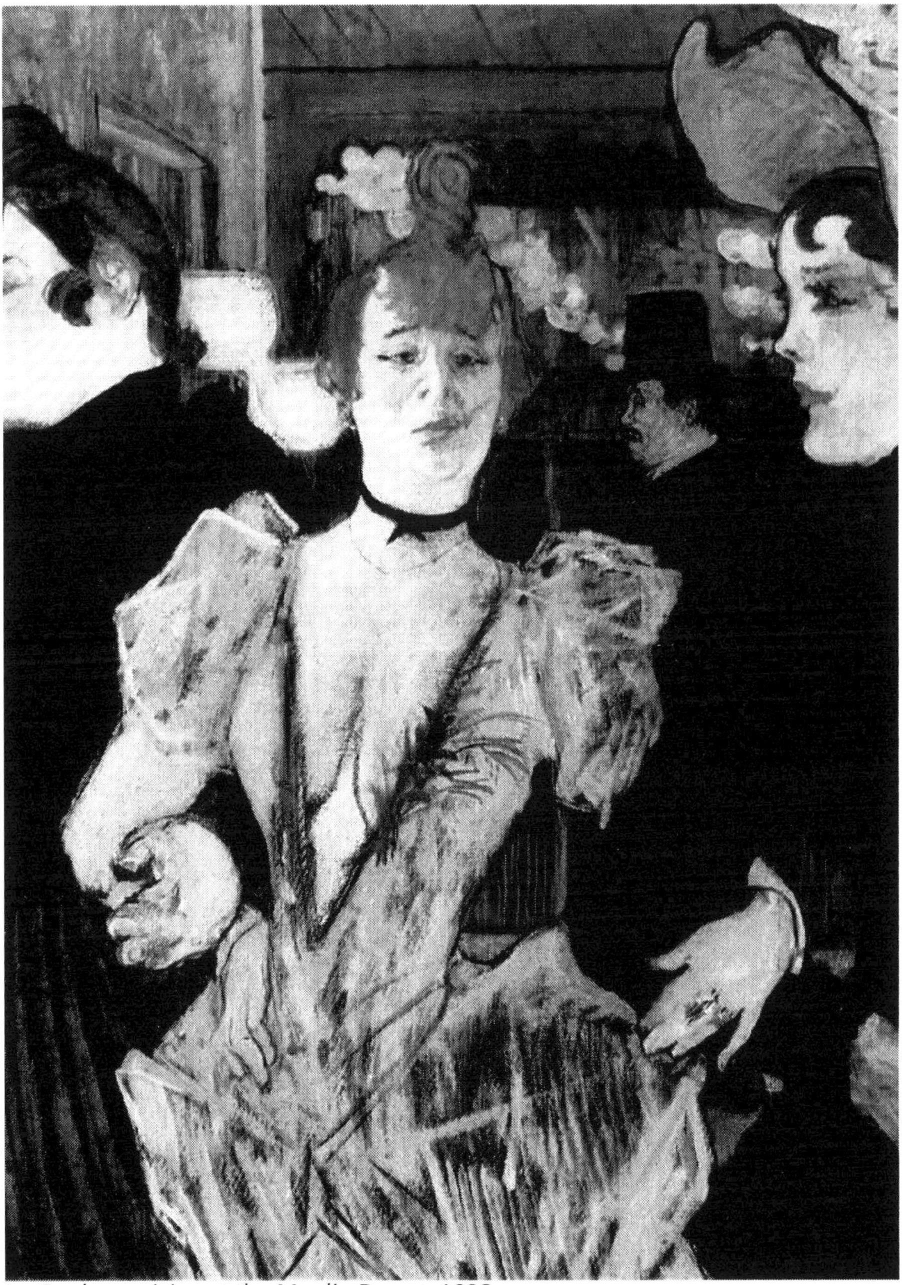
La Goulue arriving at the Moulin Rouge, 1892

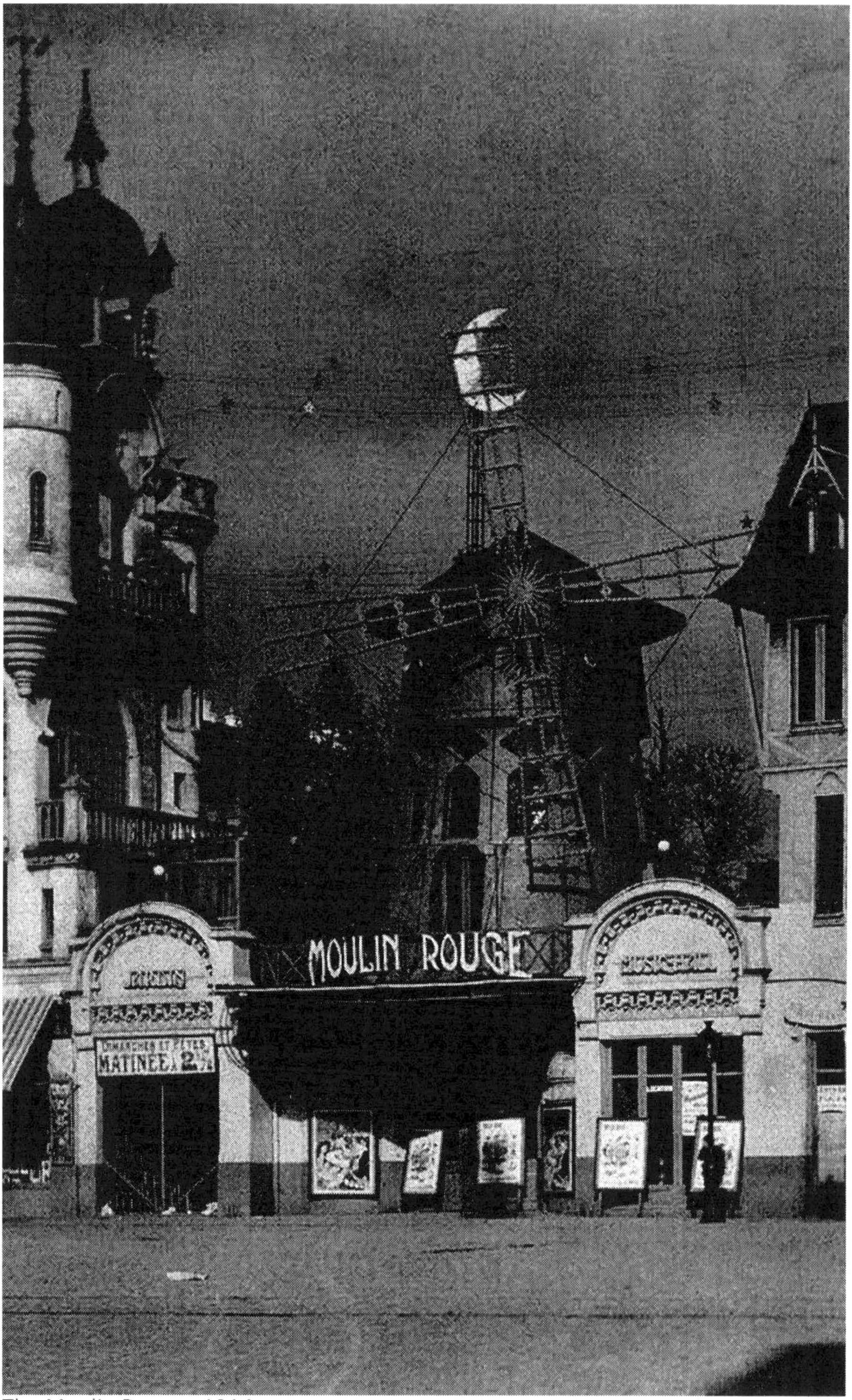

The Moulin Rouge , 1914

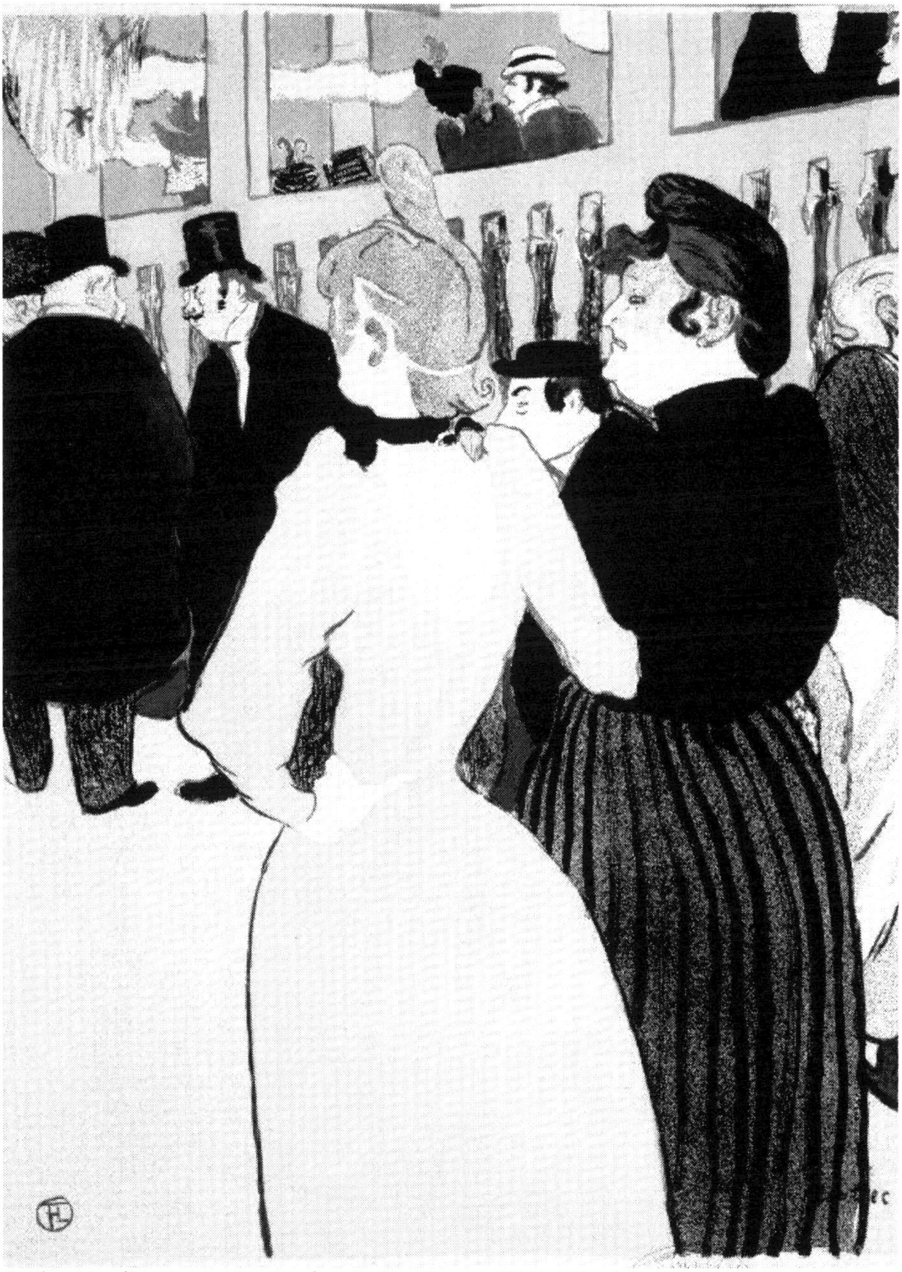

At the Moulin Rouge: La Goulue & Her Sister, 1892 | Touluse-Lautrec

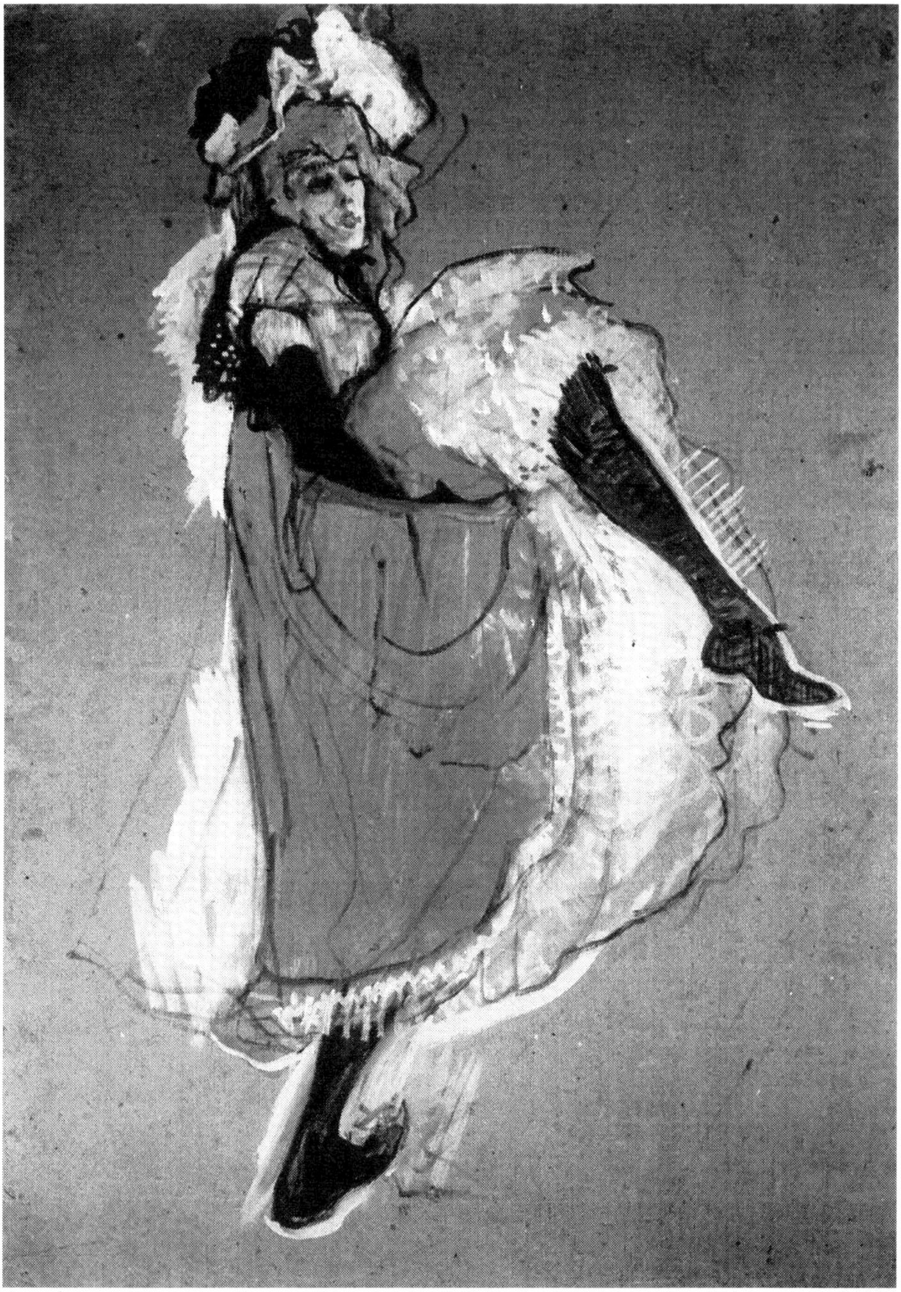
Can Can

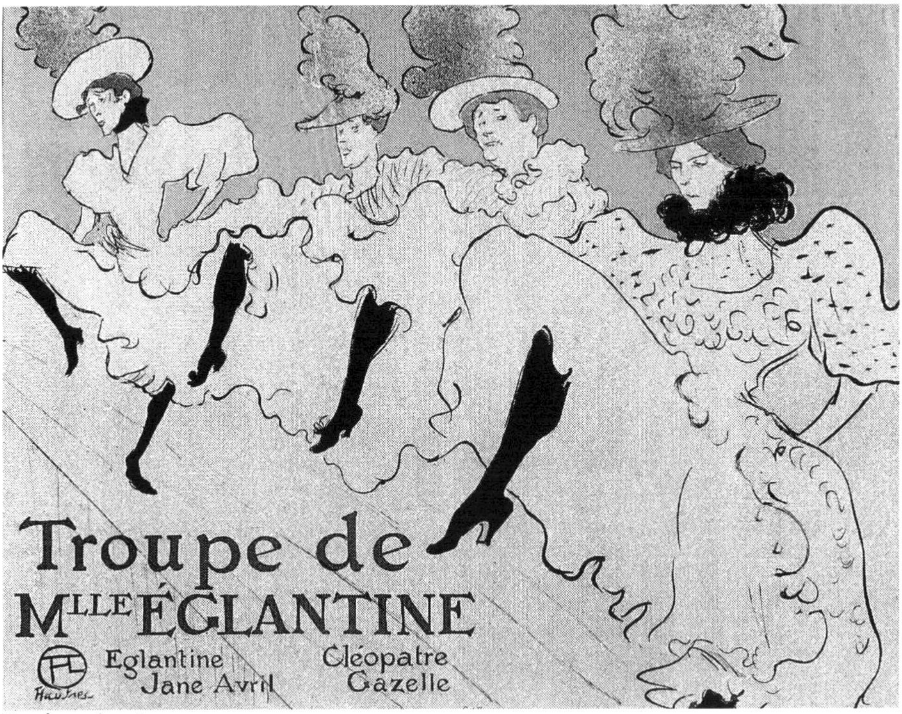

Touluse-Lautrec

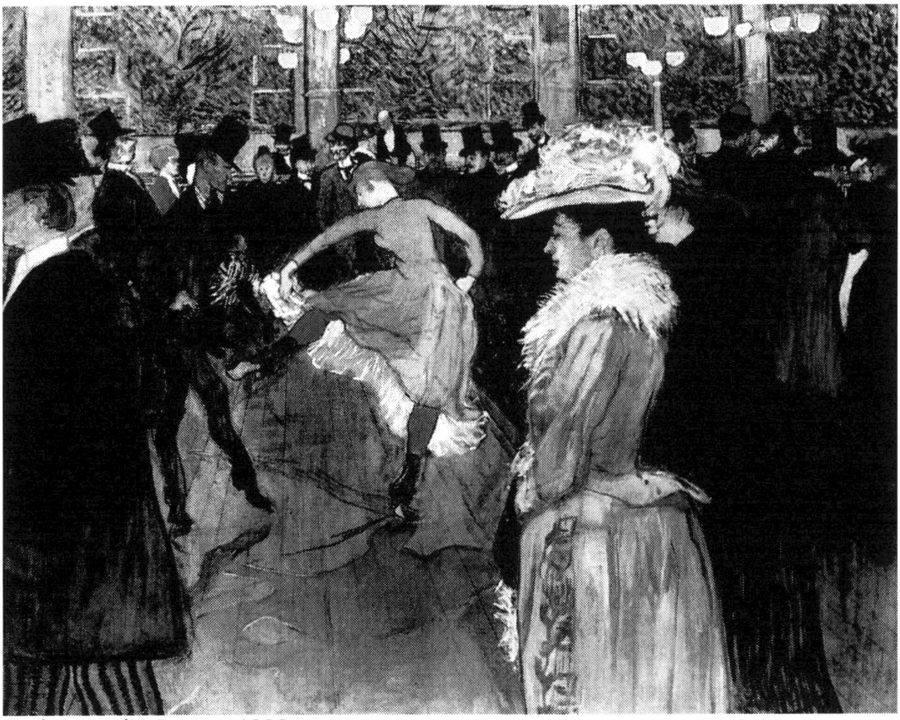
At the Moulin Rouge, 1890

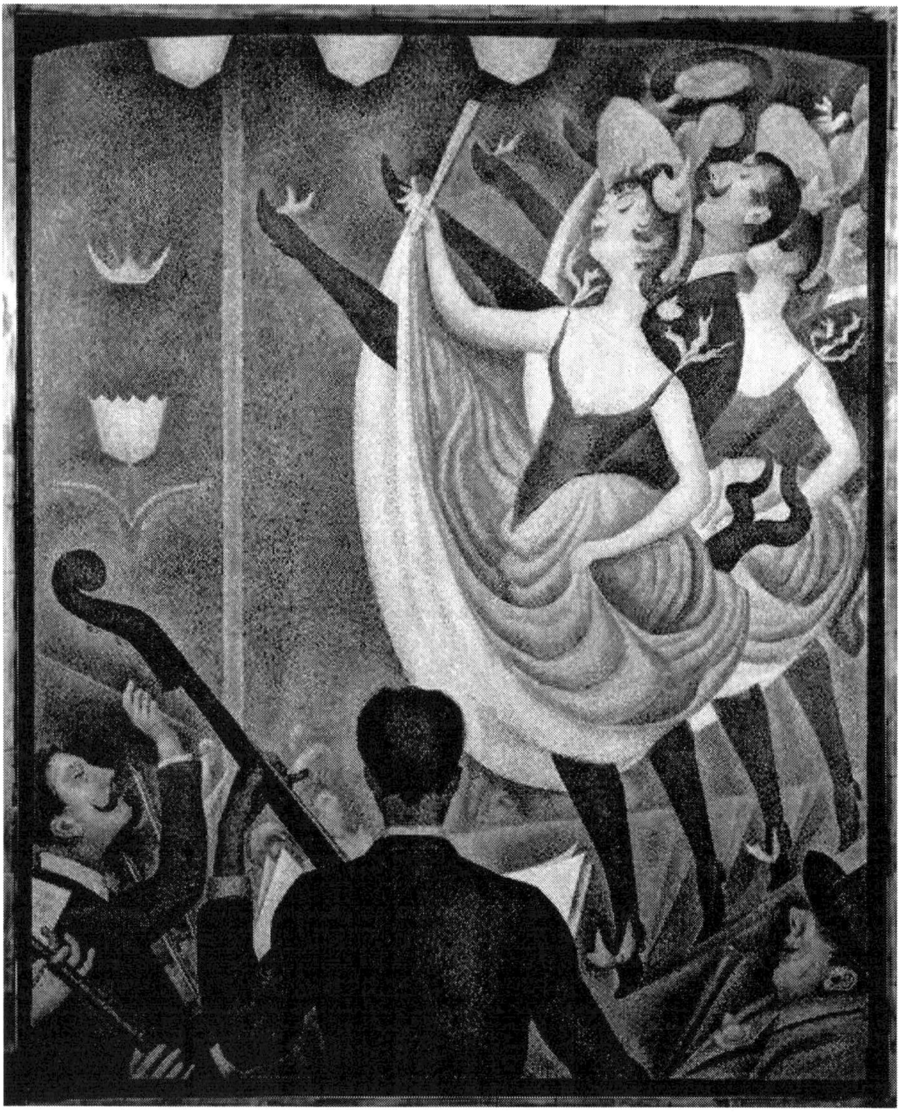

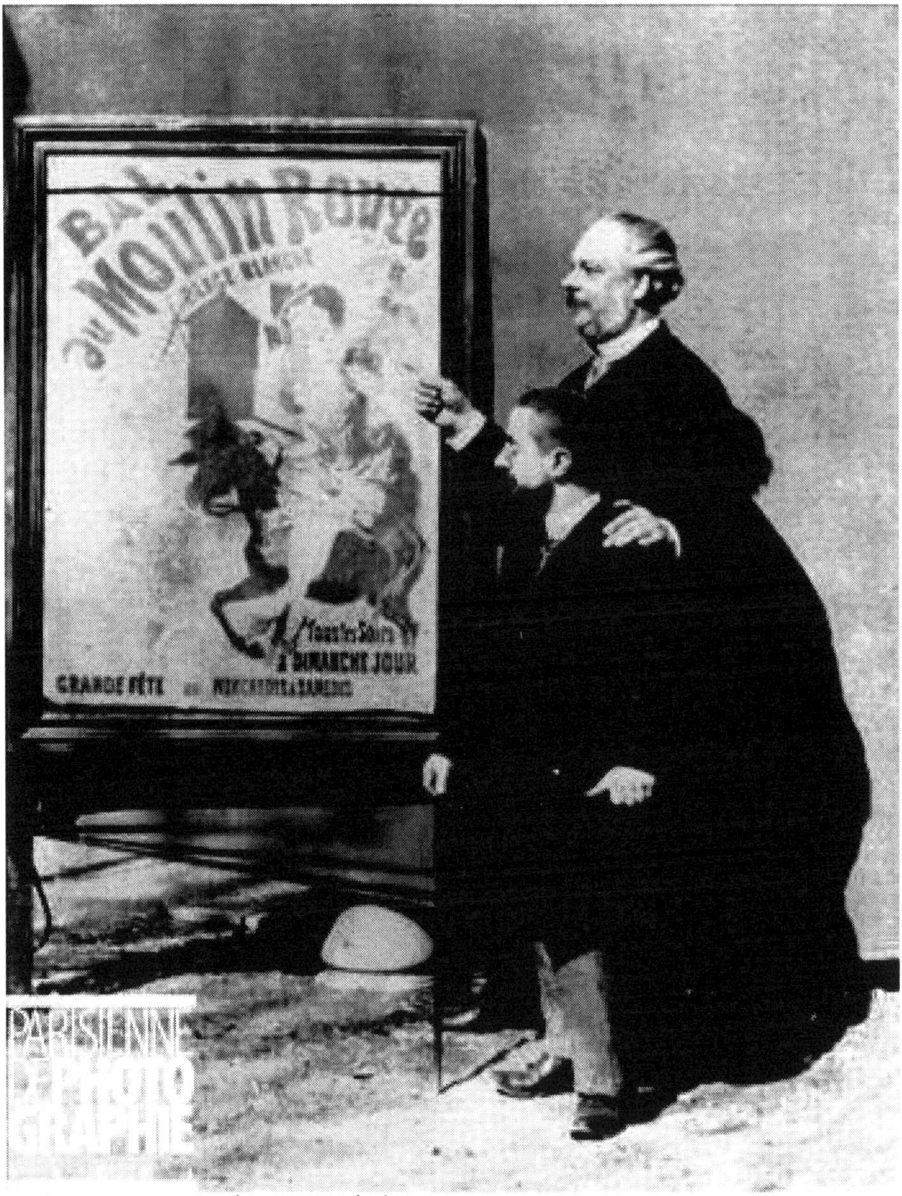

Toulouse-Lautrec and Mr Tremolada

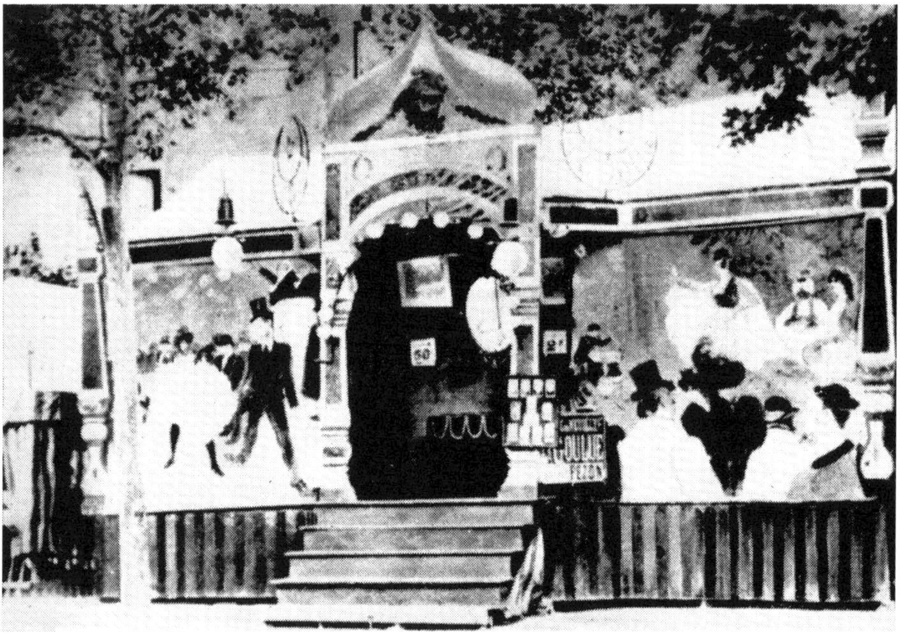

1895

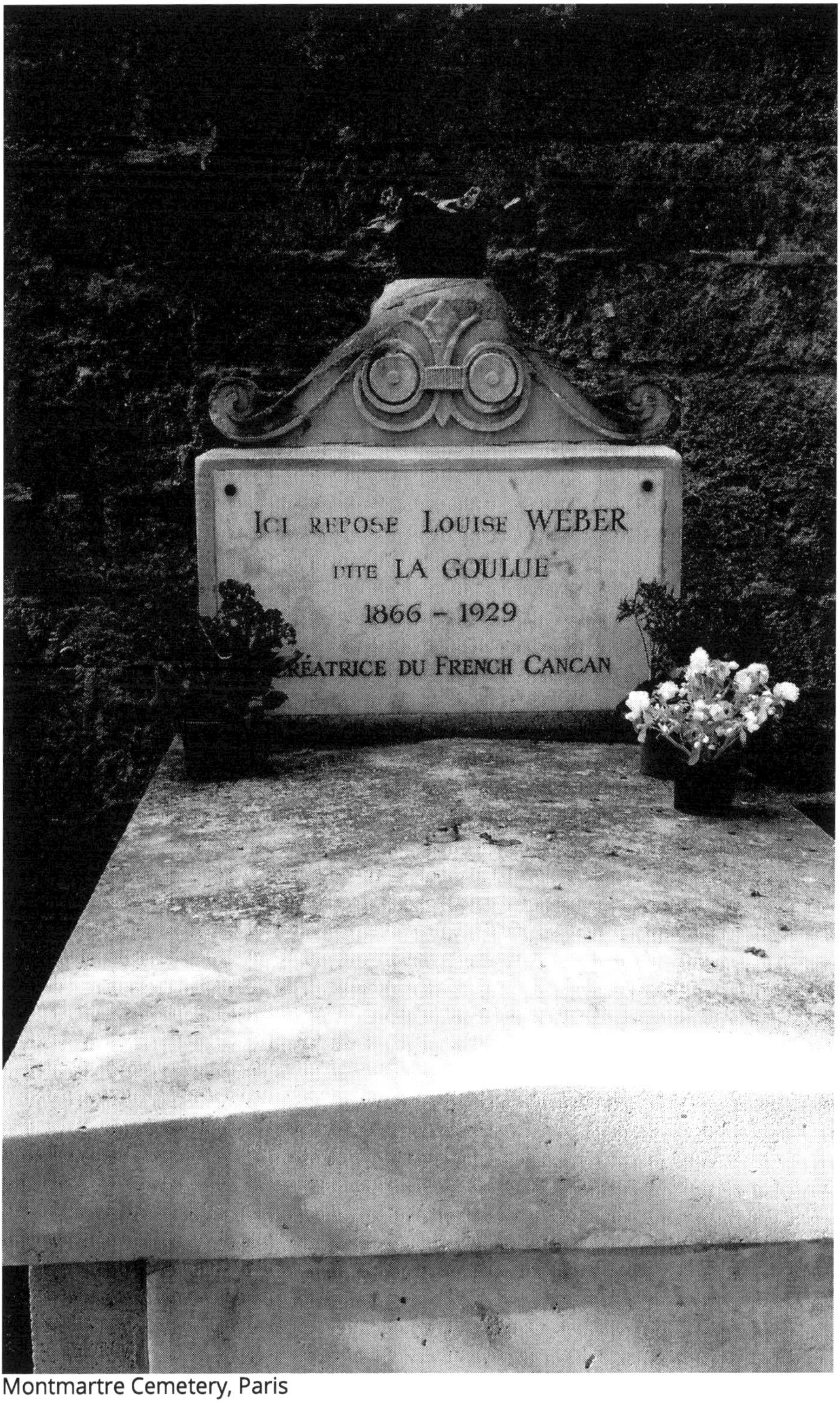

Montmartre Cemetery, Paris

ARTS IN THE STREET

-XIII-

After six years spent at the Moulin Rouge and fifteen doing the cancan, La Goulue changed her life and moved away from Montmartre. It was a new beginning, at least she thought it would be, for a new life as an artist. During the Belle Époque, the fun fair drew a considerable number of Parisians and foreigners out for a good time in the capital. The acrid odor of the menageries, the biceps of the wrestlers and the striking presence of the wild beast tamers—another name given to the job of training them—thrilled the society ladies and entertained the tarts. It was a popular fair, but a place where all the social classes would meet: high society that came to slum around at the crowd-drawing attractions, bourgeois, employees or workmen looking for simple forms of entertainment or strong emotions, all rushed over to that ephemeral city of painted canvases and planks, both brilliant and sordid, a universe of illusion, sensuality and excitement.[1] Each fair had its schedule, its rhythm, its space.

At Eastertime the Gingerbread Fair opened; it stretched from the Place de la Nation till the Cours de Vincennes. This pedestrian fair took place from spring to autumn. Then popular fairs set themselves up during the festivities on Vaugirard, others did so at the Invalides. In June, Neuilly took over. These ambulating artists moved to Saint-Germain-en-Laye, then transported their stalls in September to the Parc de Saint-Cloud.

---

1. Christiane Py, Cécile Ferenczi, *La Fête foraine d'autrefois. Les années 1900.* Éditions La Manufacture, 1987.

After the Celebration of the Lion in Belfort came Montmartre in November, and the season ended at the Gobelins and La Villette.[2]

La Goulue had just invested her savings, namely the equivalent of seventy-seven thousand euros today, in a fair stall that she would set up and take down according to the schedule of holidays or local popular events. Accompanied by several supernumeraries, she installed the arts on the street by exhibiting herself in a costume lined with sequins. Concealed under opaque veils, her body revealed her pregnancy only partially. Louise decided to no longer have recourse to "La mort aux gosses" (Death to the Kids), the nickname of an abortionist from Batignolles. How many times had she entered the back shop of the wine merchant on the avenue de Clichy? Her memory erased everything concerning her visit to this fifty-year-old bread carrier who in less than three years aborted four hundred girls and women...[3] On the Boulevard Rochechouart, she met a fortune teller. The swarthy face of the latter, lit up by two golden pupils, radiated freedom. A scarf hid part of her ebony-colored hair. The fortune teller's engaging smile and soft voice overcame La Goulue's mistrust. Paris boasted a large number of soothsayers of all conditions and charging different tariffs. At the fairs, they were called somnambulists because their predictions were made in a state of hypnotic sleep. Some of them interrogated the tarot cards, the crystal ball and the lines of the hand. The organizers of popular fairs suspected them of exercising a doubtful and dishonest profession and rejected them in the name of morality. Holding a contrary opinion, journalists supported these merchants of happiness who, according to them, were more dangerous in their dwellings than at the fair... La Goulue's heart began beating a little faster. After consulting the different cuts of her tarots, Karina announced to her the birth of a son, but also some vexations, probably a lawsuit. La Goulue shrugged her shoulders, caressed her belly, then pulled out her chest with a satisfied air, even though she avoided, at present, the clairvoyant woman's gaze. Nevertheless this

2. "La fête de Neuilly" (1940): dynastie des Pezon, dompteurs; François Bidel; hippodrome de la porte Dauphine; le funambule Castanet; La Goulue, etc. Neuilly Revue Henri Corbel, May 1901 in P. Jarry Topographie de Paris, XXXIII, p. 99, Bibliothèque historique de la Ville de Paris, part of the catalogue of the general collection I (Ms I to Ms 721).

3. Louis Chevalier, *op. cit.*

goddess of the flesh was rather proud of the carnal consequence of one of her casual encounters which made up her adventurous life.[4] Once she returned home, La Goulue was not surprised to encounter the postman who had to hand over to her, after she signed for it, a letter from the law courts. She restrained herself in order not to kiss it! Karina's voice was omnipresent: "You will know vexation and happiness!" On opening the envelope, her face lit up even though she should have shown discontent. The fortune teller was right... La Goulue would go back to the courtroom: it was Oller who reproached her for practicing disloyal competition by continuing to dance outside of the Moulin Rouge. While the envelope was burning up in the wood stove, the future mother reflected on her new outfit that would charm the president!

-XIV-

Her voice perpetually hoarse, the new fair entertainer harangued the crowd while handing out leaflets: "Tent no 1, *Great Attention*! The public was invited to come see the celebrated dancer La Goulue, the idol of Montmartre. Her show was even more extraordinary than Nini-Patte-en-l'air in Berlin!"

Her belly dance numbers were renamed "Danse de l'almée." (Dance of the Almah). It was Jules Roques who offered her the first oriental dance costume during a naturalist ball. La Goulue transformed herself, by turns, into a snake, a salamander, undulating and hissing with her belly against the ground, then picked herself up while directing all eyes towards her well-rounded rump. She swayed her hips, her waist oscillated and arched. She became a wave in singular ebb and flow movements. La Goulue created a new number with her troop.

A decoration for her stand could serve as publicity for her; she wrote to Lautrec...

April 6, 1895
My dear Friend,

I will be at your place on Monday, April 8 at two o'clock in the afternoon. My stand will be at the Trône; I am located as you enter to the left,

4. Georges Montorgueil, *op. cit.*

I have a very good spot and I would be very happy if you have the time to paint something for me; you will tell me where I must buy my canvases, I'll give them to you that very day.

La Goulue

Lautrec did not forget his friend and, in an act of solidarity, agreed to paint for her two large panels meant to be hung up outside of the tent and easy to roll up and store without fear of damaging them. The canvas was rough, the colors were inexpensive, but they bore witness to the prestigious past of the famous dancer.

The panel was divided into two parts: *La danse au Moulin Rouge* paid homage to the couple of inseparable dancers that La Goulue and Valentin le Désossé formed. The queen of the quadrille concluded her dance with a thrust of her buttocks and continued with the splits whereas "Valentin's legs stiffened and spread apart in a grotesque attitude."[5]

To better reinforce the anthological character of the scene, Lautrec depicted Jane Avril there, with an immense feathered hat on her head. The lighted garlands referred back to the imagery used at the time, when people marvelled at these new lighting effects within the framework of popular merrymaking.

The panel on the right, *Moorish Dance or The Almahs*, evoked the present of the dancer who was attempting a new career. The Moorish character of the belly dance was popularized by the World Fair of 1889. The Almah show that took place in the Egyptian and Moroccan pavilions and combined eroticism with cheap exoticism was considered a real attraction. Hence La Goulue's decision to launch her new career as a popular fair artist.

In the center of the poster: La Goulue, with her leg raised high, does a "foot in the hand," a figure of the naturalist quadrille and not at all a Moorish dance movement! She is accompanied by "oriental" musicians sitting cross-legged, one of whom was perhaps Aïcha with whom she had slugged it out… From her platform the dancer dominates the public gathered at her feet. Aïcha, whose first name was really Emma, saw the light

5. Paul de Lapparent, *Toulouse-Lautrec*, Les Éditions Rieder, 1927.

of day in 1876 in the trailer of her circus artist parents. Her father from Morocco was of Berber origin and her mother was born in a town in Piedmont in Italy. Emma would give birth in 1895 to a girl named Line, the future parent of la Môme Piaf (The Piaf Kid) …

A few people are watching the show and turn their backs on the spectators. Henri and his friends, frequenters of the ballrooms in Montmartre are reunited one last time to pay homage to the dancer: Paul Sescau, the nostalgic piano player, whose thinness inspired so much fear in the painter that he promised himself to "cushion his death," Maurice Guibert, the representative of a famous champagne firm and a connoisseur of Parisian places of ill-repute, Gabriel Tapié de Céleyran of the red sideburns, a notorious reveler, a first cousin and accredited confidant of the painter. Jane Avril, called "la Mélinite" (The Explosive One) is in the company of Toulouse-Lautrec. His silhouette is so shrunk that he barely reaches her shoulders… The presence of two writers, Oscar Wilde and Félix Fénéon, in a milieu that was foreign to them, could be explained by the painter's current life. The interest Toulouse-Lautrec showed for Oscar Wilde drew attention to him from the literary world. Henri went to London, met Oscar Wilde who was accused of homosexuality, then produced from memory a watercolor showing his face worn out from fatigue. In May 1895 he illustrated an article in *La Revue Blanche* (The White Revue) devoted to the defense of the writer Félix Fénéon. The latter, editor of the revue, would espouse the painter's cause and write insightful comments on his work. Fénéon's hatchet profile presented curious similarities with that of Valentin le Désossé…Fénéon underscored this resemblance by commenting from afar on his presence on this popular fair panel:

> Without posing for the painting, it was I whom they saw in the soft little felt hat, rubbing elbows with Oscar Wilde in the foreground among the curious onlookers who were surrounding La Goulue's platform, and not the Lithe one, the man wearing a top hat in other compositions by Lautrec. You will have to believe this, there were analogies between the two of us that were not flattering for either one.[6]

6. *Cahiers du musée d'art et d'essai,* 1984, no. 14 (Luce Abelès avec la collaboration d'Isabelle Cahn).

For a two-year period the oriental concert was set up first of all in the midst of the festivities in Neuilly, then the troop went off touring in Le Havre and other areas. La Goulue made some changes in the show. It was interspersed with Spanish dances including a wrestling number. Her sister Victorine, who in the past had been her dresser at the Moulin Rouge, became the cashier and would welcome the spectators who made the effort to see the former cancan dancer performing the belly dance along with the splits... There were eight women accompanied by a pianist who received castanet blows to his head if he had the misfortune to play too fast! In her intimate diary, La Goulue wrote:

> I danced alone... the dancers did their Arabic dances. I appeared in the middle of the concert. At that time people knew me as a dancer. [...] All of the tarts came down to see me. For decorations there were the paintings by Toulouse-Lautrec that represented the Moulin Rouge [...]. That caught the crowd's attention. That stand had class.

The tour was brutally interrupted in Normandy. Prevented from going on by increasingly frequent contractions, La Goulue returned to the capital, leaving her troop in a lurch in Le Havre. The dancers were compelled to have recourse to a justice of the peace to get the star to send them money from Paris in order to cover their return ticket. Displeased, the public clamoured for the famous queen of the quadrille who had left to take refuge in her Montmartre neighborhood...

If Louise put her career aside, she continued her social activities with her new lover and neighbor: Simon Colle. Exit Raymond with whom she thought she had conceived her child that was about to be born. Thus, on December 28, 1895, she attended with a group of spectators brought together in the Indian room of the Grand Café du boulevard des Capucines, the projection of moving images captured by the Lumière brothers, photographers from Lyon. Before her dumbfounded eyes, the wall came alive as though by magic. The sequences were linked and, even though she was bored stiff watching the working girls leave the Lumière factory, she applauded the trick horseback riding lesson. Some memories of the Fernando circus came back to her. Her heart was pounding harder in her chest, she was feeling the first pains of childbirth that were digging into her entrails. Louise let out a little cry, a hot liquid flowed between her legs. A cab arrived quickly to bring Simon and the future mother to the hospital doors.

The next day, at nine in the morning, Louise Weber gave birth to a boy named Simon-Victor. On taking him in her arms, she thought again about the Gypsy of the boulevard Rochechouart and smiled at the little angel. She was living at 14 rue de l'Écluse. A few streets separated her dwelling from the Moulin Rouge. According to her, the newborn was apparently the son of a prince, but it was Simon Colle, a popular fair artist, who would recognize him at the Public Records Office. When she betook herself in turn to the city hall of her district, the clerk there inscribed under the mention "the mother's profession": choreographic dancer. La Goulue felt like moving away from Paris in order to get to know her child. For a year, she would live off her investments and withdraw to the countryside. Accompanied by a nurse and her best friend, it was in the Camargue that she raised her little Bouton d'Or (Gold Button), the nickname she gave to Simon Victor, that reminded her of Gabriel Pierné's lyric fantasy.

> I had purchased a house in the country in Cacharel, and I lived there for one year… I lived off the investments from one hundred thousand francs. I had bought city bonds that I deposited at the Bank of France and the income of which I would collect every six months […]. I washed my clothes myself. I ate peaches and pears because they were in abundance and the little house was covered by extremely beautiful white roses and camelias.[7]

But La Goulue was getting restless, and Bouton d'Or did not sufficiently fill the void of her days. La Goulue often found herself impatient dealing with the sulking character of the child. Louise was far more a lover than a loving mother. Simon would be brought up by a nurse until he was fourteen months, then bottle-fed until the age of reason. In her Memoirs, Louise expressed her fear about her son's mercurial temperament. Simon-Victor would not profit from an accelerated schooling

7. Excerpt from Louise Weber's diary, *op. cit.*

method. Created by Mademoiselle Bonnefois, this circus school geared to travelling children was set up in her parents' former stall, the former panorama of crime! Louise wanted the best for her son and so confirmed his registration in a boarding school in Courbevoie. Only when he reached the age of twelve would he live with his mother and make the rounds of the popular fairs in the family caravan. The mother-son relationship was not the most serene imaginable. What did the son reproach his mother who loved him in her way? No doubt the fact that she took better care of his cousin Louis, Victorine's son. Simon-Victor did not manage to find a balance in dealing with a flighty mother who, by turns, evoked princes who had courted her, or lived with memories of several lovers among whom a certain Raymond seemed to stand out from among the others. This was the man whom she had loved for his elegance and beauty, with whom she had had continuous quarrels during the five years that had preceded his birth. Moreover, after proclaiming often that he was the son of a prince, she added in her Memoirs, when depicting the said Raymond: "I think I had my little boy with him." Simon-Victor was stifling in his boarding school. He was jealous of the boy who bore the first name of the kings of France and who was brought up as such by his own mother!

> My sister Victorine is a colossus, she can be seen at parties. [...] Above all she has a cute boy Louis whom I brought up until the age of twelve. The day he was born (in 1886) I was dancing at the Élysée Monmartre and they asked me to come for the birth. So I brought my friends with me. The nursemaid was ready. And we carried off the little one in his wool blanket and shipped him up to the Butte Montmartre where he received good care. My sister Victorine was alone and would not have been able to bring up her little Louis, but despite everything, she would come and hug him when the spirit moved her. Now he is grown up and is a handsome guy. He is distinguished, kind, and liked by everyone... He is the king of the French healers in Belgium. As for me, I have a little twelve-year-old boy, a passenger. He has his mother's temperament. He likes women a lot and tells me that he will get married soon...[8]

8. *Ibid.*

This son built up resentment and unearthed some memories when later in life he made his mother cough up money to mop up his gambling debts. For the moment, La Goulue was still yearning for action. All perked up, she wished to return to the stage. A village festival, the music from a merry-go-round acted on her like an electroshock. She decided, on impulse, to return to Paris and forget life in Cacharel.

> The next day, I got dressed and forgot country life, I took the first train to Paris. I sought out Fauvette and asked her to do a quadrille to be presented at the Casino de Paris. The directors Monsieur Bornay and Monsieur Desprez engaged us for six months…

A few years later, in 1912, She confided in Verneuil, a journalist at the *Gil Blas*. The latter wanted to devote an article to Simon-Victor who had just saved his mother's new business partner, Jackson the wild beast tamer, from a brutal death. The article was titled: "The Son of La Goulue." She evoked her maternity and her return to Paris:

> When the little one was born, I retired to the countryside, at the water's edge. A little house, some chickens… I was going crazy… One day, a merry-go-round arrived with its music… It was playing tunes that revolutionized me. And the next day, I ran for it, I returned to the Moulin…[9]

La Goulue took out a subscription to *L'Industriel Forain* (The Industrial Stallholder), a newspaper that connected the different members of the corporation. In issue number 342, during the week running from the 23rd to the 29th of February, 1896, she printed a little add where she indicated that her stall was up for sale:

> Stall comprising the equipment of the **LA GOULUE** Theatre, 9 metres in width by 7 metres in depth with gas fixtures. The whole in **GOOD CONDITION** - Electric projection lamps with revolving discs from the Maison Moltem. Contact Monsieur Colle. 14 rue de l'Écluse. Batignolles.

9. *Le Gil Blas*, July 18, 1912. In actual fact, La Goulue seemed to have forgotten the Casino de Paris.

For three months the announcement reappeared periodically, then stopped. La Goulue changed her mind. It was only in 1900, under the pressure of a jealous husband that she would sell her multicolored panels to an administrator of Lautrec and Degas, Doctor Georges Viau. They were resold at an auction at Druot's in 1907, during a posthumous sale, and became part of a private Scandinavian collection before being bought back by a merchant who broke them up into eight pieces, thinking he could get a better price that way.[10]

The provocative and ambiguous quality that she breathed into her performances contributed to La Goulue's success. Her almost animal sensuality combined with a rascally air drew her fair neighbor, Adrien Pezon, who was ogling her from the corner of his eye, then with both eyes when she appeared to him dressed in her almah costume. Despite the extra kilos that she kept after giving birth, La Goulue was still appetizing and revealed very alluring charms. As for her, La Goulue found the man to her liking and thought that to possess, in the short run, a personal menagerie would also be a good investment. There was one obstacle: the widow of old man Pezon who still held the purse strings, but La Goulue was certain that she would get her way. Adrien was a handsome man with an expressive and sympathetic physiognomy. His distinguished manners and meticulous appearance were the very opposite of the classic image of the carnival person. This lover of literature expressed himself correctly in a soft voice and polished language. His education was superior to that of his colleagues; it was true that his father Jean-Baptiste Pezon had entertained other ambitions for him outside of popular carnivals, but destiny decided otherwise. Adrien studied at the Louis-le-Grand lycée and obtained a literary Bachelor of Arts, but "Like father, like son," as they say, and the young graduate chose to embrace the profession of wild animal tamer. The Pezon family had made a name for itself in the capital and notably the personality of Jean-Baptiste did not go unnoticed in the circus milieu:

> With his lion-like profile framed by a short frizzy beard, his eyes sparkling with fleeting glimmers, his long, curly black hair, his ears embellished

10. In 1929, the very year La Goulue died, the canvases were bought by the Louvre Museum which put the ensemble back together again. At present they are the property of the Musée d'Orsay (The Orsay Museum).

> with gold rings like a Gypsy [...]. In front of the crowd assembled during the parade, he showed the face of a scarred Saracen and when he spoke, one imagined hearing the vague rolling of pebbles of his native Lozère. Pezon really looked like a leader of wolves.[11]

The World Fair of 1878 established his reputation as a great gladiator.

-XV-

> An odor of doughnuts and fries was floating in the air. The wooden horses, the cafés, the stalls, the lotteries, the badge games, the billiards, the wrestlers' arenas... all this dazzled the eyes, stunned the gaze of the onlookers. The travelling entertainers, men, women, children, musicians wriggled about on the platforms, screamed their lungs out until the crowd deigned to climb up the stairs to their huts. The racket never stopped. Now it was a drumroll, now a solemn sound of a bell that could be heard, the habitual ways of drawing the customers' attention. [...] As though in a dream, water sprites and almas charmed the sensitive souls with their graces and talents, even though their origin was the furthest possible from oriental, whereas thoughtful spirits much more interested in observation found satisfaction in the anatomical museums [...] Each man carried in his heart a dormant Tartarin. One had to believe this to explain the presence of so many visitors at Marck or Pezon's place where they had come specially to admire the rather peaceful kings of the Atlas and the Bengal tigers who seemed rather annoyed by the loud and detestable music they were obliged to listen to. The festival at Neuilly was reaching its climax. Parisians of Paris, rejoice![12]

To make the show even more attractive, the most unusual visits to the cages were organized. Music Hall and fair artists were in turn invited to enter the felines' dwelling. One of the most singular visits was from the torso man Kobelkoff who confronted the lions under the protection of the trainer Robert. The lady dancers also enjoyed an enormous success.

---

11. Christiane Py, Cécile Ferenczi, *op. cit.*

12. "La fête de Neuilly" (1940), *op. cit.*

Miss Sandowa performed a butterfly dance among the lions strongly inspired by Loïe Fuller's serpentine number. Pezon wished to receive the former glory of the Moulin Rouge amidst his wild beasts. He had inscribed in his program:

IMMENSE SUCCESS

"LA GOULUE'

The Real, the Unique in the cage of the wild beasts"

The information was rapidly circulated by the newspaper *La Presse* which, in its columns of April 3, 1899, announced:

> The Pezon menagerie, this year, has a new act, boasts La Goulue, the real, the unique Goulue who will enter the cage of the wild beasts.

Attracted to the handsomeness of Adrien and his fortune, La Goulue exhibited herself in the cage of the menagerie dressed in a black leotard, a light grey dolman with white braids and silver buttons. She managed to get him into her bed within a few days. The lover would initiate his mistress into the secrets of gladiator art.

To become a trainer is the result of a long apprenticeship. La Goulue took her new work seriously. The new gladiator acquired precise movements and reflexes, using the animals' reactions without loosing sight of their spectacular appeal. Pezon taught her the art of "petting" that did not emphasize the aggressive attitudes of the beasts but reinforced the esthetic quality of the show.[13]

The taming was done without whiplashes, without firecrackers that stunned the animals. Adrien would repeat tirelessly that the beasts memorized the brutalities to which they were subjected. It was necessary to know how to approach them, gently, without martyring them.

A few years earlier, a reporter from *Le Monde Illustré* (The World in Pictures) was astonished that the Grammont law that punished bad treatment

13. "La fête de Neuilly" (1940) *op. cit.*

against domestic animals did not protect tigers and hyenas against assaults by men. In 1898 a journalist suggested that the SPCA intervene to banish thrashings and blows with a lance done to provoke roaring.

Despite the competition from its rival Bidel, the Pezon menagerie was considered to be the most attractive animal collection in France and always drew crowds.

"From the humble lamp lighter to the Grand Duke heir, everyone took a seat there.[14]

Dressed in a Hungarian-styled dolmen with gold braids, Adrien stroked Brutus amicably once the animal made his entrance and lay down at his master's feet. After the gladiator opened the lion's giant mouth, he placed his own head between those terrible jaws. The beast remained calm. Pezon mounted him and rode twice or three times around the cage on his back. The highlight of the show was called "The Trainer's Sleep." Adrien Pezon lay down on Pacha, his large red lion from Senegal. The two lionesses, Bellone and Sultane, came over in turn to stretch themselves out on him while the other beasts, rooted in different poses, surrounded the group. The gladiator honored his contract and received a loud ovation from the crowd. La Goulue needed thrills, she was getting bored dancing among the beasts. Being considerate, the robust and rash trainer would teach her the art of introducing hyenas, wolves, then how to train lions.

In April 1899, the press spread the news about La Goulue entering the wild beast cage and her baptism by blood: two wolves recently arrived from Siberia were doing jumps from the bars in the central cage when one of them became furious, pounced on her and bit her on the thigh. Reacting to La Goulue's screams as well as to those of the terrified spectators, Adrien armed with a sharp prong succeeded in making the animal release its grip. A doctor came to administer first aid in the tamer's trailer.[15]

Unfortunately, this would not be the only accident of which La Goulue was the victim. Despite this episode, she came back, impassible, with a

14. Paul Hervieu, « Les Fêtes foraines, » Les Annales politiques et littéraires, June 4, 1905.

15. « Le baptême de sang de La Goulue, » *L'Aurore*, April 19, 1899.

crop in one hand and a whip in the other, to tame the wild beast that faced her in the cage.

After eleven months of living together, La Goulue wanted to have star billing and open her own menagerie. Her character was changing, she needed air and independence. She felt mature enough to take charge of her own business and her bellicose nature got the upper hand. On July 14, 1899, during the setting up of the fairground stall for the festival in Montmartre, tensions arose concerning the money due her. She considered herself wronged, despoiled, robbed. La Goulue resembled a pressure cooker ready to explode. Her plan had been to remain docile, to follow master Pezon's lessons to reach her own goal. Now, the student wanted to free herself from her teacher. The man was upset because he had not seen anything coming. La Goulue was acting like a spoiled and capricious child who would not tolerate any vexations. Her means of communication limited to a filthy vocabulary of several words was reinforced by violent acts. La Goulue had just hit her target. A set of keys, thrown in a fit of anger, had just given Adrien a black left eye. This conjugal incident induced the Pezon family to close the menagerie for several days and press charges. The press spread the news of La Goulue's mischief, and Adrien owed it to himself to relate his version of the facts in the papers. The handsome, sensitive and kind lover was wounded in his pride; he who made lions recoil and tamed bears allowed himself to be dominated by a little woman. Confiding in a columnist of the newspaper *Le Radical* (The Radical), he expressed himself forcefully in parables:

> There is nothing like one's native environment to awaken temperaments that are a bit savage. I will never take my lions to the Sahara. That way I will be sure of being in control. I should have suspected the same in dealing with La Goulue. She had been reasonable at the Place de la Nation, at the Gobelins and in Neuilly but when she saw Rochechouart, when she glimpsed the Sacré-Coeur, the rue Lepic and the blades of the Moulin Rouge, she changed.

La Goulue returned to her home base, on the hill of Montmartre, from which she sent a stamped paper. She reproached her former lover for having caused her grave artistic damage and having exploited her naivety! In her Memoirs, she conveys her bitterness in another way:

> It caused me pain to leave Adrien because I was really fond of him. He had an argument with Madame Pezon because she took advantage of the fact that I was her son's friend to justify never giving me a cent. I was exploited in this menagerie. There was the beginning of a lawsuit…[16]

The complaint became part of a demand for compensation to the tune of 11,000 francs to cover her eleven months stay in the lions' cage. Adrien retorted in court that he did not owe even a cent to a former employee, but that she owed him an amount covering the cost of a large cage wagon for carrying wild beasts, which brought the damages up to 5000 francs!

Several months later, in November 1899, the whole world of fun fairs witnessed the liquidation of Adrien Pezon's menagerie. The trainer was not yet ready to call it quits. The winter break would allow him to think of a new way to ply his trade. He wanted to retire to the family home in Montreuil-sous-Bois, to forget his disappointment with La Goulue, and to think about what he was already calling his "salon circus." It would be a kind of circular circus rather than extending in width. There would be tiers where spectators could watch the show and enjoy a full view. As for the wild beasts, they would be presented in the center of the ring…

A crowd of curious onlookers rubbed shoulders with the most famous animal trainers of the time: the Bidels, Ridenbachs, Laurents and Julianos. Buyers from Hamburg where the wild beast fair was held also made the trip. Sitting behind the auctioneer, the Police Commissioner Carpin scrutinized this mass of people. Adrien had asked for close surveillance because his former mistress had uttered some threats during their separation. Two policemen in civilian dress were ready to intervene in case of trouble.

La Goulue, discreetly attired in a dark dress embellished with a black fox scarf, standing in her glossy ankle boots, was there for business and

16. Excerpt from the diary of Louise Weber, *op. cit.*

not for a fight. Her eyes encountered the gaze of the police representative. She smiled faintly and placed her index finger on her lips as though to say: "Mum's the word... I'll only open my mouth to bid." Besides, by sending through the press[17] a letter signed Louise Weber, did she not make it known that she was burying the hatchet?

> As for Monsieur Pezon, kindly let him know, through your estimable newspaper, that he can sleep soundly. I have no desire to threaten his life. Fate will take care of that for me; besides I find it somewhat bizarre that a renowned trainer of wild beasts like him should need two policemen to protect him against a weak woman. He is giving me too much credit and too little to his animals. I hope that reading my letter will reassure him completely and allow our good policemen to get some rest...

The article was dated September 1899: two months after it appeared, the trainer was still mistrustful!

Adrien Pezon gave the sales talk himself and presented "the merchandise." La Goulue bought a little monkey and a young lioness that she recognized for having trained it when she was the carnival performer's partner. Proud of her acquisition, the young trainer crossed over the barrier and stroked the head of the beast that licked her hand.

The new owner of Bobby shook her purse filled with gold coins and paid cash for her purchases. Since she wished to start training the animal that very evening, Pezon's clerks went to look for a "sabot" (clog), a kind of cage with full lateral panels. A bit bewildered, the lioness changed owners.

At last, La Goulue finally realized her dream. She possessed her own menagerie. Her stall set up in four days was located a few metres from Adrien's. The trainer Laurent became her partner. On his advice, she bought from the Antwerp zoo a panther that was shipped to the Gare du Nord (The North Railway Station). Three lionesses, named Coralie, Mignonne and Talma, and the lion Négus joined and enlarged the menagerie. La Goulue made her debut entirely on her own for the first time at the Batignolles fair. Still curious to see that music-hall dancer braving danger, the public again came at the appointed times to see her perform.

17. *Le Matin*, September, 1899.

La Goulue decided to celebrate her first successes by popping champagne bottles in the cage where she offered a little supper whose outcome would require the intervention of the police force.

The former dancers of the Moulin came to greet their colleague, very proud to show them her set up: an attractively decorated caravan that she also used as a dressing room:

> The party started right way, there were musicians under contract to the house, who played with all their might. There were present the great Nana Serpolette (Nana the Wild Thyme), La Môme La Crotte (The Filth Kid) and Cricri. [...] I myself bought two hundred and fifty francs worth of champagne and liquors. I had at home six baskets of Ayalla champagne. We had a super supper. But the peace didn't last long. The great Nana began to put a leg on the table. She crossed the table on one leg. She was very big [...]. The Moulin dancers did a quadrille and they were all hanging on to Laurent the trainer who came in alone just to find his wife and children. There were complaints because of the musicians who played until two in the morning.[18]

An article in the newspaper *Le Temps* (The Times) dated September 16, 1899 corroborated La Goulue's words:

> Mademoiselle Weber was right at home at the Batignolles fair. The inauguration of her establishment was celebrated by a banquet for twenty-eight guests in her cage and without the lions present. The bill came to fifty-two francs. But according to the residents of the neighborhood the guests let out yells like wild beasts during the whole night and a complaint was just lodged against La Goulue, their hospitable hostess.

La Goulue got four fines slapped on her and another lecture from the police commissioner Carpin who threatened to close her menagerie. La Goulue simpered, turned on the charm and got herself out of trouble once again with her habitual flair.

> Everyone said good-by while hugging one another and everything was over. I continued my cage shows every night. They were sold out, we had to turn people away. This was how I began on my own...[19]

---

18. Excerpt from the diary of Louise Weber, *op. cit.*

19. *Ibid.*

La Goulue took her work seriously and braved danger in order to increase the box office receipts. Thus, she did not hesitate in making for herself a scarf and a garter with two large boa serpents.

> They were moving around me and squeezing me to the point of strangling me. There was always an attendant in the menagerie to take them off on time.

Fortunately, the two associate trainers, Juliano and Laurent, whom she signed up would come to her aid during the show. During the performance before the staff of the Chinese embassy, they were successful in extricating her, with pitchfork blows, from the claws of Bellonne the lioness before transporting her, in a faint, to her trailer. At the Festival of the Lion in Belfort, one of the lionesses decided to escape and take refuge under the trailer. Juliano the trainer managed to get her back into her cage and received a bronze medal for his heroic act. Jean Lorrain met La Goulue and was not impressed by her circus reconversion.

> The ex-star of the Montmartre balls performs now with lionesses, but cautiously, by keeping her quartet of numbed beasts at a distance with the gladiator's pitchfork. Fat enough to make the leotard moulding her body split apart, La Goulue moves within the undulation of a cabbage green train attached behind her. It is as brutally ugly as possible, but it has a rascally ugliness that would have enchanted Rops.

As night fell, the fair appeared in a luminous profusion of colored Chinese lanterns, but La Goulue was feeling melancholy under this magical canopy. Since her break-up with Adrien, she was again ready to fall in love. This thirty-three-year-old woman was still desirable, and some evenings the call of the flesh became unbearable. She could not live single for long. She focussed on José, a handsome, slender man with blond mustaches, elegantly attired in a white suit and vest from which was attached the pretty chain of a gold watch. This skillful conjurer, highly regarded in the "banquiste"[20] milieu for the adroitness with which he handled cards, used to

20. A person who extolls the merits of shows at a circus. He is a barker.

perform under the pseudonym of José Ducret at the Folies Bergères. Afterwards he went by the name of Joseph Nicolas Droxler, a vendor of nick-nacks on the boulevards, and fell under La Goulue's spell.

In her intimate diary, La Goulue relates her encounter with the man who would become her husband on May 10, 1900:

> I made the acquaintance of Monsieur Droxler at the various fairs where he sold jewelry and he was capable of running a circus stall, because not everyone can stand on a platform and announce to the public what will happen inside. He had a strong voice and was well suited to the task.

Just like his future wife, Joseph Nicolas Droxler had an Alsatian origin. Younger than her by six years, he was born in Paris on March 24, 1872.

The handsome lover with velvet eyes succeeded in convincing her to accept him as an associate in her menagerie. He found the words and the assurance to persuade La Goulue to introduce him as her stage manager and indeed, her personal secretary:

> A glance at the crowd thronging in front of your ticket office will tell you how to proceed according to whether it is composed of naïve onlookers who do not have any intention of committing themselves or rather nice people who can hardly wait for the sales patter to be over so that they can rush over to the wicket and shell out their good money there. Then you have to stop all the clowning, seize the opportunity and unleash the final galop that will get the undecided to race over.[21]

Convinced by this argument, La Goulue let herself by totally seduced by the dashing José who promised her to bring money into the cashbox. The two of them decided to celebrate the new century in their way by being wed!

-XVI-

1900! Never did a century begin with such a smiling face. It was a succession of festivities. The number 1 line of the Paris Métropolitain (subway)

21. "Where our country fairs are going II, The Barkers," *Le Petit Parisien*, 1922.

going from Vincennes to Maillot was inaugurated. The station entrances were conceived by Hector Guimard. The subway ticket cost fifteen cents.

> We started out well, in the direction of progress, of well-being, of science, under the maternal gaze of a France with swishing underwear and bulging breasts, one of them being the plowing of the land, the other the raising of animals, unless they were commerce and industry instead.[22]

"The Assessment of a Century," this was the theme chosen for the Fair inaugurated on April 14, 1900 by the President Émile Loubet. This peaceful sexagenarian with a rosy complexion nicknamed in Paris "Loubet le débonnaire" (Loubet the good-natured guy) would be the first President of the Third Republic to stay in office till the end of his mandate. In two hundred and five days, in a France that boasted forty-one million people, fifty-one million visitors guaranteed the success of this event. The entrance tickets of one franc (the hourly wage was between forty and fifty cents) were sold at tax offices, smoke shops and cafes. Access was free for soldiers in uniform. Ten million travellers used the subway to discover the work of eighty-three thousand exhibitors who were present over the two hundred and sixteen hectares placed at their disposal.

La Goulue and her fiancé took the rue de l'Avenir without being too impressed. This moving walkway, made up of two mobile platforms going at different speeds, and of a stationary sidewalk, enjoyed an enormous success. Set up on a viaduct seven metres from the ground, it ran along the avenue de la Bourdonnais and ended at the crossroads of the École Militaire (The Military School). For the less adventurous travellers there was a little Decauville train that ran along the whole itinerary but on rails. The two lovebirds took pleasure in leaping about on the road that snaked amidst the foliage of the trees, thus dominating the Fair. And what fun it was to jump from one platform to another and to laugh at certain passengers who took a tumble! The *five o'clock* having become very fashionable, José invited his fiancée to have tea in the Ceylon Pavilion, a charming colonial house. If Louise was sensitive to the handsomeness of

22. Henri Calet, *Le Tout sur le Tout*, Éditions Gallimard, 1948.

the Singhalese wearing immaculate loincloths, she was indifferent to the quality of the beverage, which nevertheless explained the success of this lovely corner of the Trocadéro. In her heart of hearts and in order not to vex José, she thought that this hot water would never replace champagne!

La Goulue seemed to be having fun, but her mind was elsewhere. Her thoughts were flying off to her Petit Touffu with whom she had explored the 1889 World Fair… She had been without any news of her painter ever since he had sent her the canvasses for her carnival stall. What she did not know was that he had come to the Fair of the Throne and that what he saw did not enchant him.

> He was so disgusted he preferred to flee. It was too painful to go over and say hello to her. Too painful, just like the pilgrimage he made immediately afterwards to the Moulin Rouge. He felt that the dancers were nothing more than the shadow of the past, as though they had all been infected with tuberculosis, syphilis or other fatal diseases. He fled from that place, too.[23]

-XVII-

Scheduled for April 26, the marriage was postponed till May 10, 1900 in order not to trouble business tied to the Carnival at the Place du Trône. La Goulue maintained that she had found her spouse and wanted to link her life to his. In her typically personal way of expressing herself she replied to anyone who wanted to listen that she knew enough men by now. And she also wanted to start a family. If she listened to her heart, she would have a child every year. And this is how she answered a journalist: "It is so good to have a large bunch of kids!" José's plans were simple because once married, his intention was to continue supporting Louise by drawing the crowds into her menagerie. And the future Madame Droxler declared:

> He is an exceptionally smooth talker, you can believe me! Even when all the other places in the fair are closed, there are always people at our stall. In his profession he has no equal. He is amazing. Can you believe that he

23. Francesco Rapazzini, *op. cit.*

> sometimes goes on tour without a cent and comes back with his pockets full: a true artist, indeed![24]

In a superb vehicle decorated with aristocratic crowns, La Goulue took her place by José's side. He was elegantly attired: an eight-mirrored hat, a white vest, polished ankle boots, buttercup-yellow gloves and the rest was in keeping, including a cane with a golden knob. The future married lady was decked out in a dress of black satin embellished with red roses on her chest. Her hat was adorned with a peony bush and vivid flowers. The guests were friends from the Carnival of the Throne: Romain Marseille, a professional wrestler, and his wife Louise, an acrobat; the Catalan Olivier, a snake charmer; the groom's mother; Berlingot, king of the fakers, and vendor on the big boulevards when the fancy took him. Louise's family was represented by her son Simon-Victor, Victorine and Louis, her nephew. Nana la Cascadeuse (the Daredevil) arrived a bit late, thereby causing a semi-disorder in the organization of the ceremony.

Set up at the back of a carriage, an orchestra of musicians coming from the menagerie, wearing revellers' hats, blew into horns and cornets. Drawn as much by the noisy chords of a boisterous music as by the bride's personality, an enormous crowd accompanied the spouses. The *populo* ran over to admire the former cancan dancer descending from her barouche. The American vehicle pulled by horses was wandering through the whole of Montmartre in front of workers who, half-amused, half-convinced, yelled out: "Long live La Goulue!" José scowled a bit. He was jealous of his wife's popularity. The carriage stopped noisily under the porch of the city hall. A bit absent-minded, the wedding party took a secondary staircase, then noticed its mistake and retraced its steps before finally arriving in the marriage hall.

The deputy mayor at the city hall of the 18th district conducted the ceremony promptly. He had to proceed with a more conventional marriage, and the brass concert that continued its bellowing under his windows obliged him to raise his voice.

The vows were pronounced, applause and a few "youyous" filled the hall. Congratulated by the assembled company, La Goulue had

24. *La Justice*, April 26, 1900.

them admire the enormous wedding ring offered by her husband. All of her ten fingers were already beringed with gold and silver. Simon-Victor was entrusted with an urn with which he took the collection for the poor.

An affable La Goulue extended an invitation to the gentleman who had just married her. "Sir, if you wished to come and have dinner with us on Sunday in the cage? Without any fuss. We would be truly honored!"

The deputy mayor's brow uncreased and, clucking, he expressed his thanks, but really could not accept! Elections were coming!

In the square of the Place Jules Joffrin, the musicians who were not able to enter the marriage hall struck up *La Marche des Petits Pierrots* (The March of the Little Clowns).

The new Madame Droxler bought out the whole stock of a merchant selling orange flowers with which she decorated the guests, musicians and coachmen inclusively. In slogan-singing the crowd clamoured for a dance in the Moulin Rouge style. Grateful to the Parisians who had taken the trouble to come in such numbers, La Goulue deigned to lift up her leg and knock off her husband's hat with her famous kick. A simple reminiscence of her first loves.

The press photographers were no doubt waiting for this moment to activate the lever on their cameras.

The ceremony as reported by Marie-Louise Véron, the correspondent for the feminist newspaper *La Fronde* (The Revolt), and dated May 11, 1900, gave the following details:

> Monsieur Droxler is a child of the circus. His parents are performers there and he himself began as a magician. He met La Goulue, fell in love with her and, abandoning his conjuring tricks, he has committed himself to the fortunes of the lady trainer and we will soon see him penetrate into the cages and work with his wife. At least this is what he has declared. As a wedding present, Monsieur Droxler has offered his fiancée...four lions and a superb tiger. This is almost a royal gift. Everything unfolded very suitably. The bride in a dress of black satin and wearing a hat adorned with pale roses looked very elegant and her groom was most properly attired, done up in his frock coat and holding a cane in his hand.

In her notes, La Goulue described that day in a mechanical fashion and forgot the consensual tone of Marguerite Durand's collaborator. Behind her façade of good humor Louise was unhappy. The marriage did not arouse her enthusiasm. In several pages one sensed melancholy and an omen of the separation to come:

> Monsieur Droxler pleased me well but I regretted the marriage. I saw myself as the master and I was not accustomed to be directed at the outset. The wedding was photographed, we were on the platform and I did not want to pose for the camera.[25]

Another sibylline phrase corroborated her states of mind:

> I had my little menagerie without a man and I didn't lack for anything…[26]

To a journalist who had come to record her first words as a married woman, she poured out her soul in these terms:

> "You know," she said, "Here I am married, but we are not fools, are we, Joseph? If we are not happy with each another we will separate."

The conclusion of the article did not lack bile:

One suspected more than a little that La Goulue had a long time ago eaten up all the honey of the honeymoon.[27]

-XVIII-

On July 14, 1902, the Parisian press reverberated with the latest fight of the Droxler couple: "A drama at La Goulue's place" (*L'Intransigeant*), "Parisian Drama" (*Le Radical*), "The Violence of La Goulue's Acts" (*Le Petit Journal*), "La Goulue's Revolver" (*L'Aurore*).

25. Excerpt from Louise Weber's diary, *op. cit.*

26. *Ibid.*

27. *La Justice*, May 12, 1900.

Since the exchange of vows, this marriage had already caused quite a stir, inasmuch as it was followed by several gun shots, necessitating the intervention of the police commissioner Carpin, but which, fortunately, led to very little bloodshed. What La Goulue called in her diary intimate little annoyances appeared in the newspapers and once again served her publicity.

> [...] No later than the day after their marriage, the husband in turn tried to take the revenge of the lions. From then on, the two spouses indulged regularly in fist fights in which La Goulue often came off worst. On Thursday evening, towards 10 o'clock, the husband burst into the trailer suddenly, demanded money to go guzzling, said La Goulue. Having made a big mistake about the qualities of her husband, who was nothing but a simple circus barker, his wife refused categorically, whereupon he used arguments that were so---striking that the indignant public wanted to rough up the brutal man. And as of yesterday morning, La Goulue filed for divorce...[28]

The lady trainer's crop no longer had a caressing handle and a strap made for passions. The husband no longer wanted to let himself be tamed. The quarrels and insults sometimes punctuated by acts of violence were followed by reconciliations on the pillow of the conjugal trailer. At those times the infernal lovers didn't have enough hands to count their horizontal encounters.

Often quarrels over material matters were the ones that divided the newlyweds. La Goulue reproached her husband for spending the household money and José would accuse her of dipping into the cashbox to satisfy her whims. What drove her crazy with rage was the malicious pleasure José took in reminder her of the rights that the Civil Code gave him over her, and notably article 213: "The husband owes protection to his wife and the wife owes obedience to her husband." Angered, Madame Droxler would use coarse language, but also would play with the trigger. Her last shooting session against her husband scored a bull's-eye. Four bullets: in the neck, the hip, the elbow and the right side. A policeman succeeded in disarming her just as she was going to shoot again. Bandaged at

28. *Le Rappel*, July 15, 1900.

a pharmacy, Joseph was then treated at the Lariboisière hospital where, after receiving an injection of anti-tetanus serum, the four bullets were removed from his body. This was not her first attempt. She had already shot at Droxler two years beforehand.

A good guy, her spouse attributed his wife's fit of madness to her impulsiveness and recklessness. Moreover, he would forgive her every time and would again take on his role at her side as the barker once the crisis passed.

Those two, despite their "I love you, me neither" kind of relationship, came to each other's rescue and assistance when each one of them had a brush with death in the year 1904.

In her diary, in a chapter titled "MY HUSBAND MONSIEUR JOSEPH DROXLER," La Goulue devoted a passage to these accidents connected to the Fairs at Saint-Cloud for her and at the Maison Blanche for him.

> When I had the accident at Saint-Cloud, my husband was the one who freed me from the claws and the jaws of the lion Négus and I did the same for him at the fair of the Maison Blanche when the puma jumped at his head and bit into his left leg. I was not the only one who pulled the animal away after it had clutched his leg. But I remained in the cage until the end of the session and I called in a man from the carnival who removed it completely.

At the beginning of that year (January, 1904), the press became more eccentric and spoke about La Goulue's famous revolver assault. Her husband repeated the story a few months later and also told how the cougar was killed by a firearm...

José's life was no longer in danger. With her hand still bandaged as a result of fighting off the animal, La Goulue continued her job while her husband was recuperating. This required courage, but business had to take precedence over emotions. The bloody scene unfolded before her eyes as though in cinemascope: the orchestra was playing a wild cake walk[29] whereas the beast, enervated by the music, was moving around the trainer

29. The cake-walk was a dance performed by slaves in the south of the United States. It imitated the dances of the white owners and its name probably came from the cake offered to the winning couple of dance contests.

in all directions. She could see again José's conquering face as he threw the crop to the back of the cage. Her husband stationed himself in the middle of the ring in front of the puma's open jaws. Everything went very fast, the sharp claws sinking into José's head and throat, the screams of the spectators. Then came the unequal struggle between the animal and those who came to help the unfortunate man who had fainted in his blood. After having intervened a first time and been bitten on her hand, La Goulue managed to have the last word by pumping two bullets at point blank range into the animal's cranium. The doctor called to the wounded man's bedside counted no less than a dozen gashes. The puma's corpse was tied up in a canvas and thrown under the platform. La Goulue worked the crowds while her husband recovered from his wounds. While quickly executing a few cake-walk dance steps, she invited the customers to come and see how one could be eaten up for two cents!

The accident to which she, in turn, fell victim in September 1904 could have been fatal and would continue haunting her for a long time.

She owed her life to José, from whom she was now separated, as well as to Charretier, a carnival worker who came as a reinforcement to wrest her from the claws of the lion Négus, a beast she had recently purchased from Bostock, a fellow trainer. Being impatient, La Goulue wished to show off right away without having worked beforehand with that new cat. José disagreed but capitulated quickly to his ex-wife's desires:

> We worked with him without any rehearsal. I told Monsieur Droxler: "I am going to do the splits and you will get the lion to pass over my body." He answered that I was wrong to go so fast. When one does not know the temperament of an animal, one should not be confident, especially as concerns lying down in the cage. [...] The lion stopped suddenly, threw itself at me, got hold of my stomach and dragged me to the back of the cage. [...] Afterwards, he licked my ear and took my head in his mouth...[30]

La Goulue was transported to the hospital of Saint-Cloud where she was given emergency first aid. Her carelessness could have put her life in jeopardy.

30. Excerpt from Louise Weber's diary, *op. cit.*

The press had teeth as sharp as Negus' were. As for Noël Amaudru, a journalist, he was inclined to find attenuating circumstances in favor of La Goulue's lion!

> That animal obviously does not like music and reproves the splits. [...] La Goulue's splits must have been really big to rouse Négus out of a character generally indifferent to dance in itself. They will have to invent a new aperitif.[31]

Even though she suffered agony, the trainer showed impatience. A nurse came to confiscate her clothing because, despite a fever, she wanted to get back to her stall. Her wounds were serious, she no longer had strength in her left arm because the nerves had been severed, and her left ear had also been sown back on. (The bite had come within a half- centimetre of her temple and the nape of her neck.) Her head was hurting her, she was delirious:

> I was afraid of falling asleep, I asked the doctor for a medication that would put an end to these dreadful nightmares.

The nightmare was to return to her animals that had been poisoned by ill-intentioned people, to the mange that continued to thin the ranks of her menagerie and to her marriage that had torn itself apart despite the reconciliations in the intimacy of their "chignole" (trailer).[32] There was also the fear of running out of funds and having to go back to pounding the sidewalk. La Goulue put up a good front; she joked with doctors Wassiliev and Lebour who took care of her and addressed the nursing staff in familiar terms. Fifteen days after the drama, she returned to the scene of the tragedy. Her dress of red satin embroidered with gold and stiffened by blood was exhibited, like a relic, at the entrance to the menagerie. With her legs turned to cotton and despite intermittent fevers, she returned to her place among the wild beasts. The loss of income and the fact that lemonade had

31. *Le XIXe siècle*, September 18, 1904.

32. The circus people preferred to use the terms "caravane," chignole" or "verdine" rather than "roulotte," all meaning trailer.

replaced her champagne obliged her to leave the nursing establishment prematurely, and she explained herself in a few words:

> I was too bored at the hospital. Monsieur Droxler, my husband, took care of me extremely well and got me out of the hospital. He was very attentive at that time [...] There were people crying in front of the menagerie, others inside were speaking with me and beseeched me not to enter the cage, they gave me money. Since there were no funds left, it was necessary to go back to work...[33]

A nurse came to give her morphine injections, and La Goulue biting on her quid, went back into the cage and worked with a panther that was docile towards her. Luck returned on the final Sunday of the fair: the box office takings were good and she was able to get back the awnings stored at the pawn shop, as well as a chain and a watch. Snug in her bed, La Goulue fell asleep reassured, with part of her recovered jewels hidden under her pillow.

-XIX-

On February 20, 1904, the Bal Tabarin opened its doors at 36 rue Victor Massé, in the neighborhood of Pigalle. Its creator was the composer and conductor Auguste Bosc. Ever since the Moulin Rouge transformed itself into a concert theatre, the establishment committed itself to perpetuating the memory of the naturalist quadrille.

> There would be no place here for the crumpled little faces of the Butte, for the anemic little girls, for the gutter cats, for the low-cost rotten ones, for the wallet snatchers. If any of them show up, they will be thrown out![34]

The man who directed the balls at the Moulin de la Galette and the Élysée Montmartre enjoyed great popularity, and he counted on his notoriety as well as on the quadrille to draw the foreign clientele visiting Paris.

33. Excerpt from Louise Weber's diary, *op. cit.*

34. Louis Chevalier, *op. cit.*

At the Tabarin, they danced to the rhythms of the moment: the cake walk and the mambo. The pleasure guide of 1913 specified that the prettiest demi-mondaines frequented the ball. The columnist added that one could participate in competitions that were far more entertaining than those of the Agrégation (State Exams): calf, shoulder, leg and ringlet contests... Obviously these games were simply the pretext for offering the beauties of the house to a rich, well-to-do clientele.

Bosc called on Jane Avril but also on La Goulue to ensure the authenticity of the cancan. La Goulue returned to the stage in this hall conceived in the Art nouveau style and decorated by the frescos of Willette. The newspaper *Le Gaulois* (The Gaul) announced in its columns that she was abandoning the *conjugo* (spouse) and her menagerie. Bosc proposed that she create, within his walls, a national cancan academy.

Despite her separation from her husband, La Goulue did not completely abandon her menagerie. The box office returns were meager and she had to feed her animals. Simon-Victor replaced José. The newspapers announced her divorce, but that was not the case at all. The Droxlers separated by mutual agreement. The former dancer returned to the chahut that she had illustrated in the past. The lessons were open to the public and drew a curious crowd between five and seven at the Bal Tabarin. Every evening, La Goulue's pupils profited from the afternoon lessons and their choreographic frolics brought joy to the elegant audience. Bosc's excellent orchestra was more incomparable than ever and La Goulue's national academy was the pleasurable focus of the aperitif. The whole of Paris was dancing at the Bal Tabarin.

-XX-

From 1910 onwards, the public was losing interest in circuses, menageries and theatres putting on spectacular shows. Carousels and the chahut dance were the new fashion. The circus barkers turned to new types of employment, they bought lotteries, candy stalls and merry-go-rounds when the state of their finances allowed it. It was the beginning of the decline of our trainer who, bloated, aged, could no longer project an illusion to her public. An Indian ink sketch by the painter Van Donguen is cruelly and movingly truthful. In the light one notices the eye half-closed, the tear at the mouth, the pointed chin doubled by a fold of soft flesh spread over the flounces of her blouse. Her leg-of-mutton sleeves made her appear even heavier…

It was also in 1910 that she opened the doors of her stall to a young man of twenty-two with slicked-back black hair answering to the name of Francis Carco. The bard of Montmartre appeared to be under the deadly charm of this woman who was almost nothing more than the shadow of herself.

> When I met La Goulue at the fair she was an old woman. Age, however, hardly mattered. She had that pallid complexion, those warm pupils whose gaze was dilated by pleasure; those splendid legs, that carriage, that attitude, that avid and dissolute expression that were pursuing me despite myself. The light, the odor of the acetylene lamps added an undefinably tragic and inalterable something to the intensity of memory. One thought about rainy evenings amidst the hubbub of the merry-go-rounds. […] I almost experienced dizziness from it all. Like the effect of a magical spell, the pitiful stall on the trestles of which this heavy, tired, heavily made up, hoarse gossip exhibited herself was transformed into a kind of palace…[35]

La Goulue was only forty-four years old; her blotchy face retained the scars of the accident of which she had been a victim in July 1904; with her bosom bulging out of her loose blouse, she could no longer create illusions. The bottle became her best friend, and in the evening she would come and plunk herself down on the seats of Montmartre's pubs. Nevertheless, she wished to allay suspicions as she always had, remaining dignified and proud, even though she again had to leave at the pawn shop the few jewels that remained from her past life. The words of the lecturer and man of the world André Fouquières corroborated those of Carco. He depicted La Goulue in rather coarse terms and compared her unhesitatingly to a misshapen creature with drowned features and an empty gaze:

35. Francis Carco, *Mémoires d'une autre vie – Bohème d'artiste*, Éditions du Milieu du Monde, 1942.

> I saw her in her trainer's stall at the Neuilly fair, a distressingly poor show. Balking at the slightest exercise, the beasts themselves looked as though they had been acquired on the cheap. It required a considerable effort of the imagination to convince oneself that there had once been, thronging around this woman, the most brilliant sophisticates of the era, that the Prince of Wales had come up to Montmartre one evening to see her frolic about in the racket of the brass.[36]

Yet, in the twilight of her life, a man with white sideburns came up to see her again. Elegantly attired in a morning jacket and top hat, he wore a flower on his lapel. It was with tears in his eyes that he observed this tired trainer, indifferent to the world that surrounded her. But when their eyes met, La Goulue reeled and had to hang on to a guardrail to prevent herself from falling. What was happening between these two beings whom everything separated but who were reunited by simply looking at one another? La Goulue, whose face had become livid, pronounced a few unintelligible words. The show was over even before it had begun! The old man made his way through the crowd and mounted the few steps leading to the stand. Removing his hat, he took the hands of this woman he had known, in times gone by, and kissed them. La Goulue preceded this former lover who held her delicately by the arm and had him enter her stall...[37]

La Goulue's hut was composed of a simple little enclosure closed off by planks, of a palisade arranged in a rectangle where a lion cub was stretching out in the sun while growling softly. A completely red calico band was hung up with these words: *Madame La Goulue is here*.

Disappeared, the canvasses that related the dramas of the popular fair menagerie; burnt, the relics stained with blood...

"Enter, Enter, barked Simon-Victor. You will see what you have never seen before...Come see the training of the lion Ménélik! The work of La Goulue! Ménélik trained in freedom!"

---

36. André de Fouquières, *Mon Paris et ses Parisiens – Pigalle 1900*, Éditions Pierre Horay, 1955.

37. Canyameres Ferran, *L'Homme de la Belle Époque*, Les Éditions Universelles, 1946, according to the account given by the wife of the painter Jean Cardona.

A sparse group of people entered to see a fat lady in a black leotard and a coat of purple velvet opened at the side that afforded glimpses of the opulent shapes of a formerly beautiful girl. An asthmatic orchestra tried to fill the gloomy silence that surrounded the platform. In a hoarse and tired voice, Madame La Goulue announced that her lion cub was the son of the lion at the Jardin d'acclimatation... An old man had just thrown a bale of straw in the arena on which he lay down. The young beast came to join him and had fun... La Goulue presided over these frolics then went around to collect the meager receipts in a beef merchant's money bag and recommenced her smooth talking for "the new suckers" who were listening. La Goulue knew that the public could sense she was going down the drain. What embarrassed her were not so much the crude jokes about her physical appearance but above all her inability to gather up enough money to buy milk for "Baby," the lion cub's nickname...

What had become of the time when La Goulue, dancing at the Élysée Montmartre, "Small, with a baby rose complexion and in good shape, thrust her pearly shoulders out from her largely opened blouse, and her mischievous head surmounted by golden hair, of which the heavy twisted form rolled up high resembled the crest of a helmet?"[38] La Goulue had remained faithful to her helmet-like coiffure, but the Princess of the chahut, so lively and nimble, had become a prematurely aged stout woman.

At the beginning of the general mobilization, La Goulue sold the frightened, cunning Ménélik, who suffered from rickets, to the trainer Auguste Laurent and the menagerie was thus reduced to two porcupines.

-XXI-

With the declaration of war the Montmartre of roguish pleasures lowered the curtain. As of August 2, 1914, the day of general mobilisation, the theatres, cinemas and other music halls closed their doors. The real reopening began after the battle of the Marne, with the return of the Parisians and the blessing of General Gallieni who proclaimed: "A city without shows is a defeated city." In actual fact, poverty was preying upon the little artistic

38. Eugène Rodrigues-Henriques, a lawyer and art collector quoted in *Le Moulin Rouge en folies.*

world and it was in their interest that the order of November 23, 1914 foresaw the resumption of performances. Short films called "war news" and patriotic programs were put on in certain theatres and concert cafes. With its streetlamps painted in blue to avoid being pinpointed by enemy aircraft looking for targets to hit, the streets of Paris took on a sinister appearance...

La Goulue was eking out a living by selling gingerbreads, candies and safety pins. Her cheap goods were contained in a modest basket. Her days unfolded according to the rhythm of news about her son who, mobilized in September 1914, went to join the 17th Infantry Battalion on December 19 of the same year. The photo by Charles Lansiaux immortalized the scene with the following caption: "The Class of 1915. The Recruiting Board. Madame La Goulue embraces her son who is approved to serve his Country." On that day, Louise presided over a stand selling patriotic cockades. The personage of "La Goulue" gave way progressively to become Madame the widow Droxler. José died not during the war, because he was exempted in 1894 from military service for cardiac hypertrophy, but at his mother's dwelling in the fourteenth district. A few tears ran down Louise's face but were rapidly dried! A little widow's pension would be allocated to her. Money was the obsession of this woman who was always afraid of not having enough. A little gangster snatched her purse where fifteen francs were hidden, but what she grieved for above all were the lost letters of her son wounded in front of Notre Dame de Lorette.

Louise indulged in drink to forget her solitude and the stories that were circulating about her Simon-Victor. She was supposedly the grandmother of a little Marthe, born on October 24, 1914; her boy had seduced Adeline Perruquet, a cook who came from the Aoste region. Simon did not recognize the child. Was he informed of her birth? That same year, he was living with Germaine Jullien, a pretty redhead born on March 15, 1896. The girl was fickle and enjoyed the pleasures of life. It was normal for her age, she said to herself, shrugging her shoulders. Taking advantage of a furlough, he married Germaine on February 29, 1916 at the city hall in the 9th district of Paris. The two fiancés were minors but obtained through an authentication act the consent of the two parents for the bride and that of Simon Colle for the groom. Louise Weber was reported absent, without news of her whereabouts,[39] on the marriage certificate. Did Simon want to protect himself from his mother's anger or was it the bride who did not wish to have a drunk at her wedding? The number 11[40] issue of *Carnet de la semaine* (Notebook of the week), a literary, political and satirical gazette, published on July 22, 1917 a portrait of Louise that bears witness to her decline:

> Madame La Goulue hung up the canvas of a Scientific Panorama under the archway of a subway station on the boulevard Rochechouart. Crumbling and shiny under the watered silk, she appeared on the threshold of the strange establishment like a potbellied and good-natured spider. It would cost the spectator only ten cents if he were willing to let himself be devoured. Since the war, Madame La Goulue stopped fighting against lions and getting herself scratched by trainers. The lion cost too much to feed: "And then, what would I do with it in these meatless times? Without taking into account the fact that the government would not look favourably upon it. So why do you want me to show ferocious beasts, tell me?" [...] I contemplated the old woman, heavy under her corset like compressed gelatin. The passersby winked amicably at her and in their eyes there was tenderness and, indeed, deference. [...] Nor could I prevent myself from feeling an almost historical emotion in the presence of Madame La Goulue, who wore on her face the stamp of an era, and on her shoulder the scars of lions.

That same year, Simon-Victor made the newspaper columns. The permanent War Council of the seventeenth region condemned him to five years in prison and a fine of one hundred francs. The man was implicated in a forgery affair, in the use of forged documents and in provoking desertion... The son of La Goulue was also condemned on January 21, 1919 by the 5th War Council of Paris to four years of hard labor for desertion and would be transferred to a military penitentiary in Albertville in August 1919...

39. Archives of Paris, marriage certificate Colle-Jullien, number 167.

40. Heading "Le carnet des jours, page 1, Jacques et Jean, » in *Le carnet de la semaine,* July 1917, no. III, 3rd year.

-XXII-

The year 1918 marked the resurrection of Louise. In February, the daily *Le Petit Parisien* (The Little Parisian) announced on the front page: “La Goulue is dead,” then quickly denied it the next day: “La Goulue is still alive.” The news spread like wildfire in Montmartre.

Making her way into the newspaper offices, “the resurrected one” came to rectify the facts and denounce the usurpation of her identity. It was true that many dancers had been borrowing her nickname since she left the stage.

> I am very vexed that this good woman used the name that was given to me by painters in my youth because of the good appetite I had. I would bring my little basket and I would gobble up while posing for the painter Goupil who lived on the rue des Saules in Montmartre. I was always as hungry as a wolf and they were the ones who gave me the name of La Goulue and afterwards I became a celebrity of the dance: sixteen years at the Moulin Rouge and then the popular fairs where I wore my dress with an apple green satin train filled with lacework as I stood on my platform under the trees, and that dress began to turn green at the gingerbread fair. Mothers used to come with children in their arms to see La Goulue dance with all her heart and soul before the war but not as light as she had been…[41]

The newspaper editor added that despite her fifty-two years she had maintained her bearing as an animal trainer, even though she had gotten rid of her beasts at the beginning of the war. Since then, she exercised a less dangerous trade: she sold sweets at Saint-Ouen.

Another columnist wrote:

> It is thus a false Goulue who is buried in Rouen. The real Goulue never left her Montmartre but she does not regret a misunderstanding that allowed her to read the most amiable death notices. May La Goulue, then, enjoy a long life and may luck accompany the man for whose return she is waiting. Having left the main cage for the first line of fire, Weber the poilu is committing himself heroically to tame the Krauts!

41. Georges Montorgueil, “Au jour le jour, La Goulue, » news article, 1926.

Since the announcement of her demise in the newspapers, there was a stream of columnists who came to wander around in the fortifications zone, in the vacant lots between the tottering shacks and the trailers washed out by the rainwaters.

This sordid event inspired the songwriter Georges Gabriel Thenon, better known under the pseudonym *Rip,* his nom de plume and stage name. This French magazine author wrote for her a play made to measure, that was directed by Henri Varna. The owners of the Bouffes du Nord heard of her desire to return to the stage. By dint of perseverance La Goulue managed to memorize the text and wisely heeded the staging directions that Varna imposed. The try-outs were convincing and the contract was quickly signed on a corner of the table. It was with a light heart every evening that the actress left her trailer squeezed in between the Saint-Ouen gateway and the Clignancourt entrance in the heart of the large caravanserai atmosphere of the Cité Chiffonnière (Ragpickers City) to find the stage and her audience again. A paragraph in *Paris-Midi* dated April 12, 1918 announced La Goulue at the Caf'Conc (Café with live music):

> After dancing the most eccentric quadrilles on the waxed floor of the famous ballroom of the Moulin Rouge, and haranguing the crowds on the platform of her menagerie before entering the cage of an unfortunate lion weakened by age and fasting, La Goulue is going on stage. Monsieur Dufrenne to whom she had expressed her desire "to do some acting" did not hesitate in offering her this satisfaction. In the second act of the vaudeville of which the first performance will be held tonight at the Bouffes du Nord Concert, La Goulue will come and lift her leg up as she did before!

A few years later, Maurice Hamel, a features journalist and the confidant of former glories and their misfortunes, met La Goulue in her trailer. For a little banknote of one hundred cents which she would use to go to the Flea Market in Saint-Ouen and buy herself some linen to clean herself up, La Goulue who became again Louise Weber or Mademoiselle Weber for her neighbors, opened her heart about this brief theatrical appearance:

> I had another bit of a go at the craft in 1918, during the war... It was at the Bouffes du Nord... The owners were really nice people... the décor

> was a station… I came over and said: "Where is the station master?" He answered: "I'm coming to look for my equipment." "What equipment?" I asked. Then I explained: "So what? My equipment is myself, I'm La Goulue!" "La Goulue? He answered me, there is no longer any La Goulue, she's been dead a long time!" So I got hold of my legs and said: "You'll see if she is dead! There you are, here goes." And I did my little "number." [42]

La Goulue enjoyed a succès d'estime, but in the press one could read the following comments:

> This was no longer wanted. The puppet shows had new spectators now. French gaiety full of naïve joy, of contained boldness, of elegant abandon, of naively excessive impropriety had given way to savagery and black African acrobatics. And there were no longer those good-hearted coachmen of whom Xanrof sang so mischievously and there was no longer any Chat Noir, where Maurice Donnay transformed the Butte into an Acropolis, and there were no longer any long skirts that hid the delicate shapes and the exciting thicket of enchanting undergarments. […] La Goulue had died with the long dresses, and the naked women at the Music Halls had taken away her former prestige. Toulouse-Lautrec left us with an impression of this, who with Helleu's dry points and Bonnat's portraits hang up on the infinite wall of history the charming chapter of Parisian life from 1880 to 1900.

42. Maurice Hamel, "La Goulue misses dancing but poverty does not afflict her," *Comoedia*, December 12, 1923.

THE DECLINE

-XXIII-

1925 was a pivotal year, the apogee of the Roaring Twenties. Those Twenties marked the changeover of political power with two great statesmen, Raymond Poincaré and Aristide Briand who pleaded in favor of a rapprochement between France and Germany while Gaston Doumergue, self-effacing and full of affability, would preside cautiously over the Republic.

Almost two million men died during the Great War; the fiancées of these combatants called white widows renounced marriage, thereby justifying a certain form of independence.

As concerned fashions, independence and freedom made a giant stride. On the double page of the newspaper *Le Petit Écho de la Mode* (The Little Echo of Fashion), the models with slender silhouettes had their hair done like the heroine of *La Garçonne* (The Tomboy), the novel Victor Margueritte published in 1922. The creator Paul Poiret was supplanted by three liberated women: Jeanne Lanvin, Madeleine Vincent and Coco Chanel.

This young designer in his early forties, however, hung on to the past by organizing numerous parties at his home where he reconstructed the Jardin de Paris (The Paris Garden) and drew Aristide Bruant out from his hideaway. Nevertheless, even the songwriter's unforgettable refrains had outlived their time. The curtain fell like a guillotine blade on the Belle Epoque.

A new world was emerging from the ruins of 1918, defined by the Americans of the Roaring Twenties: *Les Années folles* arrived and stunned the miraculous survivors of the trenches. People moved away from the war without, however, being able to forget it. What they adulated yesterday quickly became passé the next day. The public needed to consume and spend money that was seriously devalued. Montmartre, the Mecca of festivities before the war, became a stopping place. The artists fled to Montparnasse where each one, from La Rotonde to the Closerie des Lilas, had his headquarters.

The pavilion conceived by Le Corbusier for the World Fair became the symbol of Art deco (That Fair had been decided in 1912 for 1915, but the Great War made it necessary to postpone the project for ten years). The Eiffel tower was shining under the lights of the Lalique firm. The ornamental profusion inspired by women, fauna and flora of the "Modern Style" of 1900 preceded the return to refined forms, straight lines, geometrical decors and the use of lacquer. Man Ray, Joan Miro, Pablo Picasso, André Breton and Robert Desnos opened the way to surrealism. The Charleston flirted with jazz. Josephine Baker triumphed at the Folies Bergère after having been the revelation at the *Revue nègre* (The Black Revue) at the Champs-Élysées Theatre…

In 1923 Louise returned to the Bal Tabarin where she had created the National Cancan Academy. It was in this establishment that Pierre Lazareff did his first article on the former glory of the Moulin Rouge:

> La Goulue is there, massive, enormous, in the midst of young women who appear as adolescents next to her. They look at her with astonishment and a wave of sadness mingled with fear and affection. The face of the former queen of the "naturalist quadrille" has grown heavy. Her abundant mop of hair still crowns a sulking baby mask. In profile she resembles a bird of prey as it has often been said. The downturned and mocking mouth, steel blue eyes, a charm both wholesome and nasty.[1]

Dressed in many-coloured rags, with a fist on her hip, she held in her hand, swollen by emphysema, a jointed wood snake. In a perpetually hoarse voice, she announced the show: wrestling matches between massive women in leotards. That was not in the best taste, but, as Louise remarked

1. Yves Courrière, *op. cit.*

to her new friend who had come to interview her, "it excited the public the same way that the foamy cancan underwear did."[2]

-XXIV-

After the fire of February 27, 1915, the Moulin Rouge was reborn, like a phoenix rising from its ashes. Oller yielded the lease to a music editor, Francis Salabert. The architects chosen for the reconstruction were called Thiers, Forest and Nibodeau. The façade was reconstructed identically, with the little tower and the blades of the windmill. Only the amorous millers—girl and boy—disappeared from the landscape.

Louise was wandering around in the neighborhood and could not restrain herself from watching, through the holes in the palisade of the construction site, the renaissance of the palace dedicated to Woman, to which she entertained the thought of returning. She kept repeating in her voice perpetually hoarse from too much alcohol and smoking, between two binges in Montmartre, that "if it were necessary, I would willingly do my little dance at the Moulin!" Adding gestures to words, she executed arm movements to show what her legs would do. Dancing was still working on her and arousing her body. Because she had nothing to lose and still believed in her lucky star, she wrote to Mistinguett.

January 20, 1925
To Mystinguette, artist

Please excuse the liberty I have taken to write you a note. I am La Goulue and knowing your good reputation in favor of former artists, male and female, I am recommending myself to you for a little engagement in a revue presenting my dances, because I am in a sad situation and yet I have a name and I feel I am capable of doing a dance every evening in a comedy. I asked Madame Théo if I could arrange a dance for my cousin. She gave me some help and was very pleased with me. Valti sang for me the songs "Et le chic de La Goulue aeiou (This is La Goulue's chic, wow),

2. *Ibid.*

Paulus dans les Gardes Municipaux » (Paulus in the Municipal Guards). *These days I have no luck. I would be so happy to be able to play a small role through your kindness, you would make me happy because my money runs out every month and I just scrape by.*

Please accept, Mystinguette, my sincere sentiments.

La Goulue
59 rue des entrepôts à
Saint-Ouen, Seine[3]

Miss would not answer Louise's call for help. This kind of letter disgusted her, not because of money matters (even though Mistinguett's miserliness contributed to her legend), inasmuch as she performed frequently in charity galas, but because she could see the artists whom she had known from the start of her career aging all around her. The cicadas frightened her; they reminded her of what she could have become.

The columnist and critic Gustave Geffroy, in an article illustrated by drawings by Toulouse-Lautrec, summed up the decrepitude of this generation of female dancers who had failed to anticipate the future:

> It was from there (the ballrooms of Belleville and Montmartre) that they indeed went off, all these crazy girls who descended on the city, who would burn themselves at the lights like moths. These were the ones you would find again later on, still young and alert or wilted and decrepit. [...] The latter, for the most part, would not escape the destiny that was hounding them.[4]

If Louis regretted her dancing career, she was fatalistic about her lot and did not complain. Facing her destiny, she did not know either bitterness, anger or jealousy.

> I had money, I never counted. I had lots of it, I had too much of it, the banknotes were hanging over my head during my sleep. All I had to do was pick them up when I woke up... [...] I had bought one hundred and

3. Martin Penet, *op. cit.*

4. *Constantin Guys, l'historien du Second Empire,* G. Crès, 1920.

> twenty thousand francs worth of goods and I lived celebrated, pampered, desired on all sides. Foreigners came to Paris to see La Goulue… People invited me and for a little dance step I got a banknote of one thousand francs in an envelope… I always had a blind confidence, […] I am a good girl. I always spent and I was always very generous, we call that giving what you have. It doesn't matter, when you give you give to yourself, is that not so? Perhaps you understand why I am just a candy vendor, after having been one of the most famous women in the world… I am not complaining…[5]

As though to reassure herself, she added:

> I am holding my own and I know of some who were more splendid than me but who have become more unfortunate than I am!

Louise was combatting, silently, this sluttish life that had given her so much and taken it all back. Two hours a day, in the erotic meeting places of the Pigalle neighborhood, she would sell cigarettes and sweets to the prostitutes who nicknamed her tenderly "Maman Goulue." A religious hospice established on the very spot of Bruant's Mirliton, also employed her as a cleaning woman. The small amounts she gathered allowed her to rent at twenty francs per month the space for her trailer. In her unpublished Memoirs, Louise related how, during her carnival life, she helped the most destitute even though, when her turn came to experience reverses of fortune, she found the doors closed. A fatalist, she survived all of these outrages:

> I have a little trailer where I can cook. I had installed two benches and a table long enough where there were frequently visitors. Barkers, stall boys or guys out of work sat down at La Goulue's table. Every day I would put over the fire either a horsemeat pot-au-feu in a large pot, or dry vegetables and a pork head and three loaves of bread weighing four pounds… It was a pleasure for me to be surrounded by all these good people who were in a real mess […] I found myself with my son, my animals and not one cent.

5. Excerpt from an article that appeared in 1923 in the journal *Le Comoedia* by Maurice Hamel.

> [...] I began selling tea door to door to salvage my equipment and, as it happened, I wasn't lucky... I never found friends who offered me a bowl of bouillon during the very cold days. I didn't loose courage, it helped me know life in its bad periods...

The French cancan of 1925 barely resembled that of 1889. La Goulue, Grille d'Égout, Jane Avril were replaced by Germaine Rieux, Mercédès, Daphnée, Chloé and Mimi Arnoul. The jumble of lace and the thick undergarments were still there, but the linen sock was henceforth replaced by natural silk. In a hall with an overhanging gallery, sixteen dancers dressed in evening gowns moved about in a perfectly devised ballet that the specialists called acrobatic. The chahut was no longer popular but the rhythm was still there. The public applauded and asked for more. That was the essential.[6]

6. Jacques Pessis, Jacques Crépineau, *op. cit.*

CURTAIN

-XXV-

Three cats were purring on a mouldy bench that was three-quarters sunken. A dog, answering to the name of Rigolo, allowed himself to be caressed by his mistress who promised him to return quickly. Louise looked out of the little window of the trailer. Heavy black clouds were piling up in an already leaden sky. Her hands let the curtain fall again on the only pane in the opening. This piece of moth-eaten lace that she used to throw over her head, under the rejoicing eyes of her audience, served henceforth as a rampart to hide her intimacy. Her gaze alighted on the two yellowish photographs tacked on the wall. These last souvenirs of her past life showed her in the elegant négligé of the period and in quadrille costume with lacework and complicated ruffles. The pretty chahut dancer was smiling with all her teeth at the fat, dishevelled woman covered in a shapeless and discolored dress. Scattered to the four winds were the café concert and music hall programs, disappeared were the illustrated postcards adorned in its corners with a crown, burned were the newspaper articles relating her fortune. The souvenir trunk was replaced by a box that had held bars of soap. Louise slid in there her earnings from selling nougats, shoelaces or cigarettes… The painter Gen Paul, whose real name was Eugène Paul, a true Montmartre street urchin who had always lived in the shadow of the Sacré-Coeur, remembered La Goulue in his Memoirs:

> [..] She was standing before the entrance of the new Moulin Rouge, in slippers, in the rain, she was selling caramels spread out in a box held with string wrapped around her neck.[1]

1. J.-P. Crespelle, *Montmartre Vivant, op. cit.*

Simon-Victor died far from her in the arms of one of his girlfriends. He was the only great and unique love of her life and he had given her a hard time. He was the only man she could not tame. This son came to see her only when he had to worm money out of her to satisfy his passion for gambling. She rarely shared secrets about Simon-Victor, because she strove to preserve that little bit of intimacy she still hoped she could have with him. However, she did allow herself this one comment:

> Everything would have gone well had it not been for my son who made me sick with worry! That kid gambles like the queen of spades. I had set aside, during the time of my splendor, about one hundred bags (a thousand francs). Just about all of it has gone, melted, thanks to the child's vice! But what the devil! He'll calm down.[2]

In his autobiographic book, *Bourlinguer* (Knocking About), Blaise Cendrars evoked his meeting with Louise on a winter evening. She was prowling around the *Figaro* building trying to catch a glimpse of her son who, according to her, "was working at the place." The death of Bouton d'Or, on September 17, 1922, in the town of Conflans-Sainte-Honorine, finally hurtled her towards the other side of the mirror and brought on her decline. "Come and see Madame La Goulue! The famous dancer who was the toast of Paris!" A barker tried to draw the crowd by summarizing the dancer's past. Without hurrying, without enthusiasm, visitors entered the little canvas enclosure and took their seats on the worm-eaten benches. The curtain revealed a woman in worn out clothes, sitting on a crate and drinking a litre of red wine without letting her lips touch the bottle. Once the bottled was emptied, she clicked her tongue with satisfaction, then wiped her mouth with the back of her hand and spat on the ground while casting a heavily disdainful look over the audience.

-XXVI-

Louise was famished. If she gave priority to meals for her cats and dog over her own, their pittance was equally meager. At sixty-two, she had become

2. Jean-François-Louis Merlet, *Le Provençal*, February 3, 1929.

a wreck. Alcohol had swollen her facial traits, softened up her flesh. When she walked, her belly shook, her blouse floated like a punctured balloon. Her fat nose took on a reddish hue above words that cleared off in her toothless mouth. She still possessed her little apartment clinging to the La Cigale cabaret where she could take refuge during the winter months. The zone, the fortifications, were her entire youth. She found her home on this terrain in Sain-Ouen, among the scrap metal merchants, the nameless and the classless. Even the journalists did not venture forth any longer to knock on the pane of her open trailer. Louise did not exhibit herself anymore, she continued to survive despite her misery. Dignified. Proud. During her sleepless nights she moved backwards in her mind to the time when, despite her ferocious appetite, her flesh was firm and did not bulged out over her leotard. The world had changed but the vermillion blades of the Moulin Rouge still revolved with a hypnotic movement that captivated the night passengers. As an attentive and silent witness of this Montmartre resurrection, Louise hoped to attend a performance. René Brunschwick wrote in the *Paris-Soir* newspaper on April 9, 1926:

> Could one not set aside all or part of a night's box-office take for this star of yesterday, who has remained a decent woman, and who is unhappy, not because she is impoverished but because she does not know whether the same brilliance, the same joy, the same freedom as yesterday still reigns today in this "palace of pleasure." [...] Tomorrow let the directors of the Moulin Rouge invite this poor relation to attend a performance. She will enhance its prestige and will justify this old reputation that Montmartre enjoys. Pleasure, charity, memory, are words that often drive artists on and save them.

That rendezvous took place on February 17, 1928. Louise went up to Place Blanche accompanied by Pierre Lazareff and Jean Marèze. At the invitation of Jane Aubert and in the absence of the regular star, Mistinguett. La Miss, who had gone off to the United States, left her place to that pretty dancer who led the revue intitled *Paris aux Étoiles* (Paris Among the Stars). There on stage were conjured up feminine feats throughout the centuries, from Brooklyn to Montmartre while passing through Mexico and Mount Olympus at the foot of a temple inundated with gold. Jane had her heart on her sleeve and helped the most destitute without advertising it. However, an indiscretion in the press provoked la Miss's anger. A journalist wrote that a star of the Moulin Rouge had made a gift of clothing to the Little Urchin charity. The reporter thought it right to make clear that this gift did not come from Mademoiselle Mistinguett but really from Mademoiselle Jane Aubert. And la Miss retorted: "If one listened to them, one would have to give money every day." And a malevolent tongue wagged: "And during the day, you sleep!"

Louise did not harbor resentment towards that little diva who never answered her letter. The old woman sensed that her days were numbered. She had become too heavy to continue keeping her balance on the wire of her life. The rope was distending and would snap sharply. Sitting in the first row, between her two attentive escorts, Louise listened religiously to the words of the song "Place Blanche." It was composed by Jacques-Charles and set to music by Fred Mélé and Craven. With her eyelids half-closed, comfortably seated in her red velvet armchair, she became one with the voice of the revue leader. Here was depicted a part of her own story:

There is only one on this Earth
There will never be one in England
This is no mystery
There is only one and we posses it
It is the Place Blanche and nothing less
All throng to it
{Refrain}
It is always Sunday here
And fun is in all our hearts
Where love reigns victorious
The bird on the branch
Sings of the joyous happiness
living as couples
Because lovers tenderly clasping one another
Come and embrace under the wings of the Mill
It is always Sunday here
It is really paradise

Regained in Paris
Here is where the shopgirl
Hears compliments addressed to her
All the while her mother worries
She meets her boyfriend at the metro stop
In the month of May, very sweetly
The young man gives her as a bouquet
A handful of lilies
{Refrain repeated}
Here is where the beautiful girls
Come and go, smiling and sweet
Here is where wit sparkles
Montmartre is known for its night clubs
People go there to drive away boredom
And this is why foreigners
Make their way here…

Louise Shuddered. While the song was unfolding, her mind was wandering around the streets of Clichy where she rediscovered her loves and remembered how her virginity disappeared in the arms of the little artilleryman. The shadows of the past returned and took on the faces of her beloved parents, her son… Jean was observing this thickset and rough face, with its heavy eyelids, its colored cheeks resembling a watercolor by Constantin Guys. The carriage of her head expressed something imperious but also great kindness. At the final note, Lazareff put his hand on Louise's arm, and she came back gently to reality. The chanteuse blew a kiss to Louise, then withdrew running towards the wings. She had to change for the final number. The brass of the orchestra reverberated. Louise recognized the first chords of the quadrille. Behind his standing microphone, an announcer with slicked-back hair declared; "Ladies and Gentlemen, tonight we have the immense honor of welcoming the queen of the cancan at the beginning of this century, I mean La Goulue." The old woman wondered whether she was not dreaming while fully awake. As though pricked by a pin, she simply jumped out of her armchair. Her hands pulled a bit on her dress and moved upwards to arrange coquettishly her hair which was in a bob. Her heart was pounding wildly. The murmur was deepening.

Jean made her understand that she had to go on stage. With trembling hands Louise tightened her grasp on the steel chain from which were hanging some lion claws. She considered as a talisman this last souvenir of her second career taming wild beasts. Helped by the two columnists from *Paris-Soir,* the former queen of the chahut hoisted herself up the few steps that separated her from the stage. The noise of the applause rippled in her ears. The projectors focussing on that bloated face made the sagging of her body more visible and underscored the astonishing mask of cruel femininity of bygone times. The orchestra struck up a melody by Offenbach and Louise performed three little dance steps on the side. Then she bowed to the audience, stammering a few words of thank you in her broken voice. The public, both taken aback and moved, gave her an ovation.

These little dance steps in which she rediscovered her crazy youth, Madame Louise would perform them one last time in 1928, in front of the fixed gaze of a camera. This silent documentary film in black and white was realized by Georges Lacombe, at that time an assistant of René Clair. Lasting 29 minutes, its title *Au pays des Chiffoniers* (In the Land of the Ragpickers) evoked the daily life of the rag-and-bone men population living in the zone.

This was the final walk around the ring for this tamer of a menagerie without wild beasts, of this dancer without an orchestra who had become a beggar holding out her hand only so that others could shake it in friendship.

At the end of the evening, Louise returned to her trailer with a few extra banknotes in her purse. The amount collected during the lottery devoted to impoverished stars was handed over to her. That small offering allowed her to improve her everyday fare.

-XXVII-

Louise was salivating. She had not eaten a good potato salad accompanied by saveloy for a long time! “Some saveloy, a soft piece for my cats and a veal bone for Rigolo.” On the half- caved in steps of her trailer, she was muttering out loud, just to remember the improvised list of errands with the few coins she picked up during a sale of laces on the boulevards…

Louise continued her soliloquy: "Before giving my dog the bone to gnaw on, I will cook it in water with some vegetables. That will give a bit of flavor to the clear broth that I have not stopped drinking since my setbacks..." Louise laughed heartily to herself at her play on words...[3] She tightened the woolen shawl around her opulent chest. She walked with small steps towards the grocery store. The blinking sign of the bar and tabaco place winked at her. She would willingly drink a little glass of rum to warm herself up. A few snowflakes were dancing in the sky, a little north wind had just bitten her face that had already turned blue from the cold.

Suddenly the ground gave way. Louise had just slid on the sidewalk. A passerby called for help. Louise's eyes stared at the sky. Was she going to take off for the celestial quadrille? In a murmur, before losing consciousness, she let out: "Is it already my time to go? Still, you are somebody when you have been La Goulue!"

3. The French play on words is based on "boire" and "déboires" meaning "to drink" and "setbacks." The sentence in French reads as follows: ... « je n'arrête pas de boire depuis mes déboires. »

EPILOGUE

Under an inky sky, Jeannot, his companion Sylvette and myself are reunited at the cemetery of Pantin. There is nothing sadder than this forsaken spot at the end of the world where the tombs all have the same impersonal appearance. For lack of means, our friend could not be buried according to her wishes in Montmartre. From a distance, because he is living henceforth in Belgium, Louis, the son of Victorine, sent a money order so that the body of his aunt would be laid to rest differently than in a coffin "offered" by public services and would not be carried in a poor man's hearse.

On this dirty early morning we are waiting for the mortuary carriage drawn by two wheezing nags. Among the paths of the seventy-fifth division, I can barely count ten or so people who succeed in making their way through the muddy alleys.

Among the few people in attendance: Émile Saint-Ober, an out-of-work actor who became a night watchman, Rétoré, the last king of hearts of our deceased queen and a few neighbors from the plain of Saint-Ouen. From afar, I recognize the silhouette of Monsieur Deranlot. He is the secretary general of the Circus Union who has come to represent the corporation. I think back to the fauna of the Moulin Rouge. I light a cigarette and concentrate on the article that I will write in the column of *Paris-Soir*. I strive to repress this gnawing anger that invades and dominates me. Two questions are burning my lips and I am holding myself back from screaming. Why have you not come, you who were one of her comrades, Pomme d'Amour, today a fortunate and respected publicity agent? Why are you not here, Nini Patte-en-l'air whom one still meets in Montmartre, covered in jewels and warmly wrapped up in sable fur?

The princesses of the street Mesdemoiselles Beuze and Hellengue, alias Grille d'Égout and la Môme Fromage, preceded Loulou to the grave. In an era when Paris had lightness as an emblem, so many names and nicknames have been lost in the night of time. After having appeared often in the limelight, Louise passed away miserable and forgotten. Rétoré whispers to me with his fetid breath that she was placed in her coffin dressed in her gown with the green train that all the old Parisians knew, the very same one that she used to wear during her famous quadrille and in the cage of the wildcats. I hear again as an echo Jean Lorrain's words referring to Louise, "a roguish ugliness that would have enchanted Rops..."

Jeannot puts his hand gently on my shoulder. I notice that the little cortege of close friends has approached the freshly dug hole where the coffin will henceforth lie. I listen absent-mindedly to Rétoré's little speech followed by a few words muttered by a priest who was willing to come by. I am unaware of the holy water sprinkler that the sacristan holds out to me. My hands shake a little when I take out of the inner pocket of my overcoat the little bouquet of violets bought from a lady street merchant. Without looking at the people in attendance, I murmur: "Don't worry, Louise, I have told them that you had been a good girl!" The flowers accompany the bier in which Madame Louise Weber, the widow Droxler is henceforth resting. Jean and Sylvette wave to me and I answer with a nod of the head. I want to be alone. I move away while stifling a sob. Through my tears, I make out two employees of the municipal service of funeral rites who are in the process of taking down the two crowns of pearls on one of which one can read: "To my aunt" and on the other "To our late friend, her neighbors."

Within a few minutes, the horse-drawn convoy will return to its mourning factory. The neighing of the horses combines with the croaking of several crows perched in the bare trees of the deserted cemetery. A timid ray of sun forces its way between two thick clouds but does not manage to warm me up.

After leaving Pantin, I wandered about on the boulevards like a sleepwalker. How did I find myself in front of the Moulin Rouge? Damned chance… or not! A small poster is set up at the main entrance. A spidery scrawl handwriting indicates that the place is "Closed for renovations." The mythical hall is going to become an ultramodern movie house. In this year 1929, the world is breaking up, going crazy. This is really the end of the Belle Époque and the Roaring Twenties…

UNEXPECTED EVENT!

-XXIX-

Michel Souvais, the son of Marthe Perruquet (the daughter Simon-Victor Colle refused to recognize), wrote to the mayor of Paris to transfer Louise Weber's ashes to the cemetery of Montmartre.

Her new tomb was inaugurated in March 1992, with all the honors of the Republic of Montmartre and the associations of the Butte as well as the Moulin Rouge.

Under the gaze of the national and international presses, two thousand people attended the ceremony, including La Toya Jackson, the star, that very year, of the show *Formidable* at the Moulin Rouge.

To this day, no square nor street mentions yet the name of our queen of the cancan.

ACKNOWLEDGEMENTS

Monsieur Jean-Luc Phéau-Ricau, Director of Communications of the Moulin Rouge,

Madame Isabelle Ducates, Director of the Society of History and Archeology of the 9th and 18th districts of Paris-Le Vieux Montmartre,

Messieurs Alain Larcher and Claude Bena, in charge of the Archives for Researchers,

Monsieur Jean-Michel Bück, Member of the Friends of Old Montmartre,

Monsieur Christian Capdet, President of the Historical Society of the City of Clichy.

The Historical Library of the City of Paris,

The National Library of France,

The Archives of Paris,

Remembrance and Cultural Affairs Service of Police Headquarters,

Thank You to Julie Daniel, the first reader at the Éditions Le Rocher, for her enthusiasm and confidence,

Raphaël Delpart for his friendship that honors me,

Nathalie de Broc, Karine Lebert, Jeanne-Marie Orliaguet, Daniel Doudoux, and Jean-Paul Lefebvre-Filleau for their precious advice and support during this long but memorable writing adventure,

Thanks to Louise for having accompanied me during my research…

LA GOULUE'S PARIS HAUNTS

Bal Tabarin: A Parisian cabaret situated on rue Victor-Massé in the 9th arrondissement at the foot of Montmartre. It was founded in 1904 by the composer and conductor Auguste Bosc. It enjoyed an immediate success and all Parisians in the know flocked there to dance accompanied by various noises: car horns, gunshots, and to participate in masked balls and flower battles. It was replaced by a supermarket in 1966. La Goulue directed the National Cancan School there.

Batignolles: A neighborhood in the 17th arrondissement of Paris. It is bounded on the south by the Boulevard des Batignolles. La Goulue frequented the thermal baths in that area whenever she noticed an increase in her girth. She even took her pet dog with her to enjoy the experience.

Belleville: A working-class neighborhood mainly in the 20th arrondissement of the city, and one of the strongest supporters of the popular revolt known as "La Commune" in 1871. Geographically it is not far from the area called Montmartre.

Place Blanche: A square in the area of Montmartre, famous for being the place where the Moulin Rouge nightclub is located. In her heyday La Goulue was the undisputed queen of the establishment.

Rue Caulincourt: One of the main streets in the area of Montmartre in the 18th arrondissement.

Avenue des Champs-Élysées : One of the most famous and glamorous streets in the world, with the Arc de Triomphe at one end and the Place de la Concorde at the other. It was already famous in La Goulue's time.

Chaussée d'Antin: A street in the 9th arrondissement of Paris. La Goulue frequented an elegant boutique there to purchase the lace petticoats for her cancan dances.

Clichy-La Garenne: An industrial commune in the northwestern suburbs of Paris. In La Goulue's time it was a rather poor, working class neighborhood that the so-called "right people" did not frequent.

Place Clichy: The only point in Paris where four arrondissements, the 8th, 9th, 17th, and 18th meet. A very lively square today as it was in La Goulue's era when it had a much more working-class atmosphere than now.

Boulevard de la Tour-Maubourg: A very high-class artery in an extremely high-class neighborhood of the 7th arrondissement. It was as much a prestigious address in La Goulue's time as it is in the 21st century. One of the lady's wealthy admirers lived there.

Montmartre: Situated in the 18th arrondissement, Monmartre is a large hill or "Butte" in French, 130 metres (430 ft) high. For this reason, it is often called "La Butte Montmartre." This hill gives its name to the surrounding area, part of the Right Bank in the northern section of Paris. In the latter part of the 19th century and at the beginning of the 20th, during the *Belle* Époque, many famous artists such as Auguste Renoir, Claude Monet, Edgar Degas and Henri Toulouse-Lautrec lived and worked there. La Goulue enhanced the glory of Montmartre since she was the undisputed star of the Moulin Rouge cabaret during the first ten or so years after it opened in 1889.

Saint-Ouen: This is a commune in the Seine-Saint-Denis department in the Île de France region of France. It is located in the northern suburbs of Paris, 6.6 kilometres (4.1 miles) from the centre of the city. It was a working-class area in La Goulue's time and remains one today. It has one of the most famous flea markets in the world and was a prominent one when La Goulue was alive. Towards the end of her life, an old and impoverished woman, she would sell candy in that area.

LA GOULUE'S HAUNTS AS A CIRCUS PERFORMER

Place de la Nation : It is a large circular space in the eastern part of Paris, and a place where many popular demonstrations begin. During the French Revolution it had one of the most active guillotines.

Neuilly: This was and remains the most elegant and expensive of Paris residential suburbs, just west of the city itself, and immediately adjacent to it.

Parc de Saint-Cloud: This is a national territory to the west of Paris and near the capital. It covers 460 hectares (1,100 acres) and is considered one of the most beautiful gardens in Europe.

Saint-Germain-en-Laye: A commune in the Yvelines department in Île-de-France and located in the western suburbs of Paris, at 19.1 kilometres from the capital. It is one of the most affluent suburbs of the city.

La Villette: In La Goulue's era, this area located at the northeastern edge of Paris in the 19th arrondissement, was not a particularly glamorous one. It housed slaughterhouses and a cattle market. In the 21st century it is an exciting place to visit. The Parc de La Villette contains fanciful gardens, the City of Sciences and Industry as well as three major concert halls and the famous Conservatoire de Paris.

Cours de Vincennes: A major traffic and commerce axis bounded on the one hand by the 12th arrondissement (the Bel Air neighborhood) and the 20th arrondissement (the Charonne neighborhood) on the other. It has one of Paris' most important markets.

GLOSSARY

Jane Avril (1868-1943*)*: Behind her apparent exuberance and the nicknames "Jeanne La Folle" (Jeanne the Madwoman) or "La Mélinite" (The Explosive One) that she hated, Jane Avril was a refined lady. Moreover, it was said about her that she was a teacher who had fallen in with a gutter crowd.

Le Chahut: This dance was a form of the can-can, a very popular, unbridled version of it in the 1840s, in which female dancers kicked their legs rhythmically to coincide with the beat of raucous music.

La Commune: An insurrection of Paris against the French government from March 18 to May 28, 1871. It occurred as a result of France's defeat in the Franco-Prussian War and the collapse of Napoléon III's Second Empire. Its proponents formed a radical socialist, anti-religious and revolutionary government which was defeated by the regular French army during "The Bloody Week" beginning on May 21, 1871.

The Decauville Railway: Used at the Exposition Universelle (World Fair) in 1889, this was a 3 km. (1.9 mile) long 600 mm. gage railway line, which operated there from May 6 to October 31, from the Esplanade des Invalides to Avenue de Suffren in Paris.

Dreyfus: In 1894, Captain Alfred Dreyfus, a career army officer of Jewish origin was accused of selling military secrets to the Germans. This accusation was totally false. He was convicted by a court-martial. He was not exonerated until 1906. The "Dreyfus Affair" caused a political convulsion in France and eventually led to a formal separation of church and state.

Léon Gambetta (1838-1882): A French statesman, and one of the most important political personalities in the first years of the Third Republic. He was instrumental in establishing free, secular education, compulsory civil marriage, opportunity for divorce and in enacting anticlerical legislation.

Grille d'égout (Sewer Grill): The very colorful and quite unflattering nickname attributed to the Moulin Rouge can-can dancer, Lucienne Beuze, by her journalist boyfriend, Henri Rochefort. This former teacher's mouth was indeed lacking one out of two teeth. Her semi-toothless jaws thus looked like the sewer grills of the era.

Grisette: This term referred to a French working-class woman from the later 17th century through the 19th till the Belle Époque, although in the process the word underwent some modifications to its meaning. In 1694 a *Grisette* was simply a woman of lowly condition, and *grisette* derived from *gris*, referring to the cheap grey fabric of the dresses she and her contemporaries wore. But by 1835 the *grisette* was defined as a working-class woman who was coquettish and flirtatious. Some combined part-time prostitution with a so-called "honest" trade.

Pierre Lazareff (1907-1972): A prominent French newspaper editor. Already in his youth Lazareff had acquired a reputation as a gifted journalist. In 1931, when he was the new editor of *Paris-Midi*, he was appointed editor of the newly created evening paper *Paris-Soir*. By combining sensationalism and human interest stories with perceptive editorial comment, he succeeded in increasing its circulation in five years from 134,000 to nearly 2,500,000. During the Nazi occupation of France he went into exile to the U.S. where he became head of the Voice of America broadcasting programs, then to England, where he directed American broadcasts to Nazi-occupied Europe. In 1945 he returned to Paris where he became the head of a new evening paper, *France-Soir*. In 1958 he entered the field of television with a news commentary that enjoyed much popularity. He was Jean Marèze's boss.

Édouard Manet (1832-1883): A major painter and engraver of the end of the 19th century. He was a precursor of modern painting that he liberated from academism. Manet is wrongly considered to be one of the fathers of impressionism. He differed from the impressionists through an art that was centered on reality. His painting, "Olympia," caused shock and astonishment when first exhibited in 1865 because various details revealed her as a prostitute.

Mistinguett (1875-1956): Her real name was Jeanne Florentine Bourgeois. She was known as the lady with the divine little legs at the Moulin Rouge. Later she would produce the kind of dazzling shows that are still popular there.

Jacques Offenbach (1819-1880): Born in Germany to Jewish parents, this composer of immensely popular operettas like *Orphée aux Enfers* (Orpheus in the Underworld), *La Belle Hélène* (The Beautiful Helen) and *La Vie Parisienne* (Parisian Life) epitomized in his music the *joie de vivre* and champagne-like effervescence of the Second Empire in France, thereby demolishing the myth of intrinsic and irreversible differences between cultures and nations. La Goulue enjoyed dancing to his irrepressible music. Wanting, however, to be taken seriously as a composer, he wrote a phantasmagorical opera *Les Contes d'Hoffman* (The Tales of Hoffman) which he was unable to complete before his death.

Le Pétomane (The Petomaniac): This was the nickname given to Joseph Pujol (1857-1945). He was a star attraction when the Moulin Rouge first opened. He drew audiences with only a bowlful of water and his rear end, producing incongruous noises that provoked their mirth.

Le Quadrille: Originating in the 18th century as a stately series of dances involving four interlinked couples, it morphed during the 19th century popular balls into a wild, improvised succession of dance steps that would eventually be called the cancan.

Pierre-Auguste Renoir (1841-1919): Among the masters of impressionism, this artist is the one who produced the most paintings based on the human face and scenes of happy contemporary life such as *La Balançoire* (The Swing) and *Le Moulin de la Galette* (The La Galette Mill). His sensual vitality and shimmering light effects can be admired in his feminine portraits and his nudes, such as *Jeunes filles au piano* (Young Girls at the Piano) and *Les Baigneuses* (The Bathers).

Tartarin de Tarascon: An anti-hero created by the French novelist, Alphonse Daudet in 1872, Tartarin, an inhabitant of the city of Tarascon, is a teller of wildly improbable tales involving hunting down dangerous animals. To prove to his fellow-citizens that he deserves his reputation as an invincible hunter, he goes off to Algeria where he manages to kill a lion. Alphonse Daudet devoted two more novels to his incredibly naïve and boastful protagonist: *Tartarin sur les Alpes* (Tartarin in the Alpes) in 1885 and *Port-Tarascon* in 1890.

Valentin (1843-1907): Nicknamed *Le Désossé* (The Boneless One or the Lithe One), this rubbery man with the elongated silhouette remains something of a mystery. According to legend he gave a total of 83,112 performances at the Moulin Rouge and was La Goulue's favourite partner. He danced for his own pleasure and never accepted a cent for his appearances, even though the Tout Paris flocked to see him. He disappeared suddenly one day without leaving a trace.

Le Grand Véfour: One of the most famous gastronomical restaurants in Paris in La Goulue's time as it still is today. It has been a meeting place for the Parisian political, artistic and literary elite for over 200 years. It overlooks the gardens of the stately 17th century Palais Royal.